HOW TO DO IT: 2

HOW TO DO IT: 2

Examinations/academia/
research and communication

Third edition

Edited by Deborah Reece

BMJ Books Editor

BMJ
Publishing
Group

© BMJ Publishing Group 1979, 1985, 1987, 1990, 1995

First published 1979, 1987, 1990
Second edition 1985
Third edition 1995
by the BMJ Publishing Group, BMA House, Tavistock Square,
London WC1H 9JR

British Library Cataloguing in Publication Data

A catalogue record for this book is available from the British Library

ISBN 0 7279 0895 2

Typeset by Apek Typesetters Ltd, Nailsea, Bristol
Printed and bound by Latimer Trend & Co, Plymouth

Contents

III RESEARCH AND COMMUNICATION

Preface

The *How To Do It* series has proved very popular, both in its regular appearance in the *BMJ* and as a series of three volumes. Some chapters have stood the test of time, being as relevant now as they were up to 15 years ago, but most subjects have moved on. We therefore thought that we should ask the original authors to update their chapters. Where this was not possible we commissioned new authors. We have included articles that have been published in the *BMJ* since the last volume was published and added chapters on new topics as they presented themselves. New authors worked hard to preserve an existing style while adding something of themselves.

Considering the old and the new articles together points up some interesting changes in writing style since the late 1970s. No longer is it acceptable to refer to all doctors as "he" and use expressions such as "the ladies' programme" for conferences. It's not only political correctness but also reflects the larger number of women entering the profession—and reading these books. But more difficult to explain is the fact that the new contributions have become more serious, their authors keener to provide a comprehensive account.

The health service has itself changed. Recent reforms have altered procedures, structures, and people's jobs. Emphases have shifted, and some topics such as audit, have grown so much that covering it in a single chapter was impossible. Doctors now increasingly recognise the importance of management, and this is reflected in the revisions and new chapters.

In the previous editions the order of publication in the *BMJ* dictated the order the chapters appeared in the books. The new editions gave us the opportunity to group the chapters together with some sort of logic. The three volumes of the series now have individual themes. This second volume covers the categories of examinations, academia, and research and communication—in fact everything you need to know to be an academically successful doctor. From the beginning (how to take examinations), through to chairing a conference, advice is abundant and sometimes unexpected. John Stokes tells juniors not to be put off by the avian characteristics of their examiners; Sir Robert Shields warns against "lasering" your audience when giving a lecture; and Richard Leeper eloquently reminds us of the "teeth, lips, tip of the tongue" progression to a strong lecturing voice. The chapters on choosing and using new technology provide down to earth information and advice. Meetings can be a nightmare to set up, and Ian Capperauld and A MacPherson provide a comprehensive checklist for would be organisers.

I would like to thank all of the contributors, old and new, for writing so well and so willingly. I would also like to acknowledge Helen Bodenham, our editorial assistant, who has revealed a detective's talent for tracking down authors, without which these books would be—well—smaller.

DEBORAH REECE
January 1995

I EXAMINATIONS

1 Be an examiner

John Dawson

It is hard work being a conscientious examiner and the task should not be underestimated. It is all too easy for the examiner to forget what an important ordeal it is for the candidate. Failure to qualify on time is nearly always perceived as an unmitigated disaster by the candidate. There is a serious loss of self-esteem and confidence. Lack of success in a professional milestone is likely to affect career prospects. Furthermore there is a prospect of increased debts as grant support and examination fees for the resit are frequently impossible to obtain. Postgraduate examinations are slightly less desperate, as failure at the first sitting is common and doesn't mean loss of livelihood.

It therefore follows that as the examiner you should be interested, alert and courteous. There is nothing more off putting for the candidate than an uninterested or a discourteous examiner.

Examining informs teaching. It is very easy to pitch the level of clinical teaching much too high and assume that the skills of taking a history and eliciting physical signs are readily acquired. The longer one examines, the more clear it becomes that this assumption is untenable.

The staging of a clinical examination is a major undertaking and upheaval for the host hospital and school. The advent of hospital trusts, the reduced length of stay of inpatients, and the reluctance of patients not only to attend as outpatients, but also to submit to repeated physical examination make the provision of a good mix of both long and short cases increasingly difficult for the organisers. Much of the burden will fall upon the host examiner's departmental

3

secretary and junior staff. You should try to speak to all the personnel involved during the examination and whenever appropriate to thank them personally for their help.

When examining in your home city it is all too easy to tack examining on to a normal day. The result is usually a hectic schedule with a constant temptation to cut corners. Examining out of town tends to be more relaxed and enjoyable not only because of the forced separation from routine professional responsibilities, but also because there is time to enjoy the unfailing hospitality of the host department.

The examination

You should arrive in good time so that you can see the clinical cases adequately, preferably together with your co-examiner. It is unfair to judge a candidate's performance unless you yourself have met, talked to, and examined the patients. Avoid examining patients with diseases or disorders in which you have a special interest; the conversation may become unreal. And remember that the candidates may have been taught things with which you profoundly disagree.

Examiners probably perform better if the morning and afternoon are spent differently, for example, clinicals in the morning and vivas in the afternoon. Spending a whole day with a relentless number of vivas is very dispiriting. The provision of alcohol at lunch time is probably inappropriate and best avoided. It can only heighten the drowsiness and ennui that may set in during a long, hot summer afternoon session of vivas.

Essay paper

If asked to contribute a question it is preferable for you to indicate what issues the candidates are expected to cover in their answer. Without such agreement, difficulties in marking are increased. For many postgraduate examinations a model answer is now a requirement and allows better discussion at an examiners' meeting when the paper is set.

All papers should be marked before the examination begins. This allows early exchange of papers, especially the borderline ones. It is very helpful if notes are made on the script explaining the reason for the mark given, especially indicating serious errors and omissions.

4

MCQs

Multiple choice questions have usually been set by a group of examiners with a special interest in this type of testing. Most examining boards already have a large bank of questions, so it is unusual for individual examiners to be asked to contribute. If you are, beware! Agreement about the wording and context is very time consuming. The practice in some examinations where all examiners have to sit the MCQ paper might fruitfully be extended to all.

Clinicals

The long case is assessed on (1) the history, (2) physical signs, and (3) the commentary, which includes an interpretation of 1 and 2 as well as further management. Most examiners regard 1 and 2 as critical; a clinician who cannot elicit an adequate history and physical signs is likely to be a liability despite an encyclopaedic knowledge of the subject. If necessary, you should return to the patient with the candidate to go over the history or physical signs under observation.

The presentation of the history is best spoken by the candidate using his or her notes as an *aide-mémoire*. In this way the salient features can be pursued and all the negative findings omitted unless relevant.

It is essential that you make contemporaneous notes about the candidate's performance, especially errors and omissions. These may be critical in the assessment of borderline candidates later.

It is also important to be present at least for part of your co-examiner's half of the examination time. Candidates frequently perform quite differently with the two examiners, and it is much easier to come to an agreed mark if you both have been present for much of the examination.

Viva

It is essential that you have no knowledge of the candidate's performance in the other parts of the examination. It may require some ingenuity to set the candidate at ease of the beginning of the viva. The heat of the moment has often induced a manic train of thought and it is essential to slow down the flow of words and restart the discussion slowly at the beginning.

Pathology pots are often used to initiate discussion. There is a considerable variation in the standard of presentation and preservation of these specimens; some are unrecognisable. The bizarre and esoteric ones are best not used. It often releases tension if the candidate is first asked to describe the specimen and identify the tissue before proceeding to identify the abnormality or pathological process. You should be looking for logical deduction rather than random guesswork.

Similarly, in a discussion of x-ray films it is important to establish the type of examination and candidates should know what preparation is required as they are likely to be ordering such examinations in the near future. The way the candidates read the film frequently tells much about their understanding. Inspired guesses, although correct, will reveal little.

The use of instruments in vivas is diminishing. However, it seems reasonable that the candidate should recognise and understand the priniciples of, and complications consequent upon, the use of catheters and intravenous lines for which they will be responsible when working in the wards.

It may be useful for you to write down a list of topics for discussion during the examination. Otherwise by the end of a long day you may be overtaken by the feeling that your total knowledge has shrunk so much it could be written on a thumb nail. A variety of discussion topics lessens boredom. It is an awful experience to examine with someone who always asks about the same topic or a very limited number of topics; although not quite as bad as working with the examiner who asks the questions you asked of the previous candidate. A good contemporaneous record of the viva and the reason for the agreed mark awarded should be made in note form.

Examiners' meeting

It is a priority that all examiners attend the examiners' meeting whenever possible to decide the aggregate mark. The notes made during clinicals or vivas are invaluable in making judgments, especially about borderline candidates. If a candidate is failed it seems reasonable that the examiner should be there in person to explain the reasons for failure.

Although the pass standard is difficult to define, there is an amazingly good agreement about the final decision on a candidate.

Examiners' report

A written report is usually asked for by the examining body and should include fair comment—both criticism and praise—about all parts of the examination, including the standard of the written answers. If appropriate, it is important to record an appreciation of department members separately. The planning and organisation of professional examinations, especially the clinicals, is an enterprise fraught with so many difficulties.

Despite all the above cautions, examining with congenial colleagues is a very enjoyable experience, more so if you leave sufficient breathing space to do the job properly without feeling pressed for time. Almost without exception the host examiner will have made your visit as agreeable as possible.

2 Set and assess a multiple choice question examination

David Lowe

In undergraduate and postgraduate examinations there can be little to equal the scrutiny candidates give to the multiple choice question (MCQ) examination. Essay questions can be set with scant regard to their wording, though of course they shouldn't be. Essay questions phrased "Write short notes on . . ." or "Discuss . . ." are usually taken by the candidates to mean "Write down everything you know about . . .", but multiple choice questions are very carefully considered by all parties. Multiple choice ("multiquestion") examinations have become widespread and generally accepted over the past 20 years.[1] There can be few of us who have not sat, composed, or organised one. This does not mean that multiple choice questions are universally admired: there are many senior academics who deplore the necessity for this style of question, but who none the less accept that it is an unavoidable, practicable way of assessing factual knowledge. For examiners there are several attractive features: objectivity; ease of scoring, especially when computer-marking facilities are available; and simplicity of interpreting the results.[2] For undergraduate and postgraduate students who have to take such examinations things are not so easy. There are different terrors from writing an essay or taking a viva examination. Candidates always protest that in a multiple choice examination some of the questions are ambiguous or incomprehensible, and it must be accepted that they are sometimes right.

Organising a multiple choice examination

Organising a multiple choice examination is less straightforward than might appear.[2, 3] You will need to think about six main points:

- the standard of the examination
- the and scope of the examination
- the source of the questions
- the number of questions
- the timing of the examination
- the quality control of the examination.

The standard of the examination is the most important aspect, from which the other points follow. You must decide what events will follow from the results—such as that a candidate will be given a prize, encouraged to continue, asked to resit, recommended to retire—and whether the multiple choice questions will achieve the necessary distinction between the worthy and unworthy candidates to allow this. The standard will vary among formative exams (which are usually in-course and may have an educative component to see how the students are doing and help them on their way) and summative exams (which in medicine are usually designed to assess competence to practise). The scope of the examination—what topics you decide are important to be covered in the exam—will be decided partly by the standard of the examination, and partly by expediency in the light of training and other factors. The standard, scope and control of an examination can be the hardest aspects of it and, unfortunately, in many instances are the last to be considered.

The source of questions may also be difficult. It is relatively easy to follow precedent and pluck multiple choice questions from an established university or royal college bank without considering whether the subjects they cover and the style they use are proper, important, and discriminant.

It is usually easy to decide the total number of questions and the proportion in any subsections of the examination. The acceptable number of questions an hour will depend on the standard of the examination and the complexity of the questions. For undergraduate examinations, a reasonable rate is one question a minute with an additional 10 minutes for every 50 questions. Some postgraduate examining bodies set only 30 questions an hour.

The quality control of the examination is a very important aspect if errors are not to be perpetuated (see below). It should be applied at as early a stage as possible. If the results of the multiple choice examination can be critically assessed before the candidates go on to the practical and viva stages of the exam, you may be able to prevent unfair elimination or disadvantage.

Styles of multiple choice question

There are many styles that you can use to set a multiple choice examination. The simplest is a list of questions that require a yes or no answer, although this is not strictly a multiple choice examination. There is the "pick one of the following" sort (also called "one from five") in which there is a question and five possible answers, of which one is right and four are wrong.

Other styles that have been used include pairing from two lists ("match each of the diseases 1–5 with the characteristic type of inflammatory cells listed A–E") and arranging a set of five choices into a logical sequence "The best sequence of investigaton, in time order, of testicular enlargement is . . ."). There is a complicated relation analysis style in which the candidate has to decide whether an assertion and the offered reason ("Mesothelioma is a characteristic tumour of asbestos workers *because* asbestos penetrates mesothelial cells") are true and consequential, both true but not consequential, the first true and the second false, vice versa, or both false. Many people find this style quite bewildering, especially under the pressure of an examination. Fortunately, it is seldom used in Britain.

The commonest format of most multiple choice questions is the "determinate response" or "multiple true/false" style. There is an introductory statement or stem followed by a choice of five options or completions. The stem and an option together are called an item, and any of these may be true or false. (Options have been called "responses" in some publications. As the stem should be an incomplete statement and not a question, its predicate is not really a response. It is the candidate who makes a response to an item.) False items are called distractors. The candidate has to decide whether each item is true or false, and in medicine is usually allowed to respond with "don't know", on the grounds that recognition of uncertainty is important for a doctor. The decision is marked as correct, incorrect, or zero.

You might consider breaking away from the "one plus five" mould. Some examining bodies, such as the Royal College of General Practitioners, have done so to good effect. This can be a simple but powerful way of cutting out useless, obvious distractors and elasticating the number of useful, discriminatory questions that can be asked on a subject. There is no good reason, other than historical usage, why multiple choice questions should be restricted to five options. Unsuitable distractors may have to be included to make up the number, and these have been shown to be poorly discriminant. Why not have three, or ten, proper options rather than padding with useless distractors? The total number of questions should be kept constant to allow comparison with previous examinations.

If you have a bank of 600–800 questions, there is an argument for making them public, as some of the royal colleges have done. It has been shown that publication of questions makes them easier to answer, and so the assessment of the examination should take account of this. On the other hand, the less able candidates will probably gain less advantage from using a book of published questions than the brighter ones.

Writing the questions

Writing multiple choice questions is a laboriously acquired art. It is much easier to advise how not to write them than to give a simple way of doing so properly. A few guidelines are worth considering. The questions should be:

- relevant
- short
- understandable
- discriminant.

That is, they should be worth asking and based on the right subject matter, be concise and clear, and differentiate acceptable from unacceptable candidates.

Data for the questions may be derived from any source; textbooks, review articles, and case reports that have a literature review are often very useful. The latest medical research is not usually suitable for multiple choice questions unless the data are widely publicised.

To compose a multiple choice question you could make a list of the points from an article that you think are essential facts or core knowledge, and then think of a stem that leads the question into the right area. Distractors are usually more difficult to invent than true

11

Example 1: An acceptable question

IgG (immunoglobulin G):

A   fixes complement.

B   crosses the placenta.

C   is formed as part of a secondary immune response.

D   triggers leukotriene production.

E   takes part in the allergic response.

Example 2: An acceptable question

B lymphocytes are:

A   phagocytic.

B   precursors of plasma cells.

C   able to carry immunoglobulin on their surfaces.

D   found in lymphoid follicles.

E   stimulated into mitosis by phytohaemagglutinin.

Example 3: An unacceptable question

Cystic fibrosis:

A   is rarely a disorder of endocrine glands.

B   is inherited as an autosomal dominant condition
    with an abnormality of chromosome 5.

C   patients have a reduced sodium chloride in sweat.

D   is not associated with intestinal obstruction.

E   results in biliary cirrhosis in 10% of cases.

Example 4: An unacceptable question

Endocarditis:

A α haemolytic strains of enterococci are the commonest bacterial cause.

B requires three sets of blood cultures to isolate the pathogens in most cases of culture positive endocarditis.

C caused by streptococci may be treated with a combination of penicillin and gentamicin.

D associated recurrent fever may frequently be due to superinfection of a valve by antibiotic resistant bacteria.

E non-bacterial causes of endocarditis are very rare.

---

items, and the mark of a good question is often the quality of the distractors. You could try substituting a similar anatomical site (*small* for *large* bowel), an attribute of a related substance or condition (IgM: A, crosses the placenta), or a recognised misconception (Testicular teratoma: A, typically metastasises to inguinal lymph nodes), but you must ensure that the distractor items really are false, and this can be very difficult.

Relevance

The questions should test important knowledge. Many medical facts fit well into a multiple choice format but may be quite unimportant in the theory or practice of a specialty. For example, in a clinical examination a question can easily be set asking which blood group is commonest in patients with gastric carcinoma, but the knowledge of this is of little diagnostic or therapeutic use. Similarly, general surgeons probably do not need to know whether corticotrophin releasing hormone is or is not a tripeptide, but might be expected to know the course of the lateral cutaneous nerve of the thigh.

The balance of topics should be checked. When an examination is in several parts and the questions are submitted by different parties it is easy for a topic to be duplicated. For example, the histopathology and microbiology parts of a multiple choice examination could ask very similar questions about tuberculosis and helicobacter infection. The medicine and pharmacology parts of a multiple choice

13

examination could easily duplicate questions on diabetes mellitus and inotropic drugs.

When the questions are taken from a bank you should check the range of topics that they cover. If the questions are chosen at random, you may be provided with 45 questions on neoplasia and five on inflammatory and metabolic conditions rather than an even spread. If the scope of the subject matter is not controlled, the candidates' marks may be impossible to interpret.

Brevity and clarity

The stem and options should be unambiguous, readily understood, and as short as possible. The stem can be a short statement or outline a clinical picture:

- Nasal polyps are . . .
- A patient who has recently returned from Africa presents with rigors. Urgent investigations should include . . .

Stems that are only one word usually need long options.[4] This is not necessarily a problem (examples 1 and 2), but there is a danger that the determinate response style of a multiple choice question can be weaselled into a set of five straight true/false questions only broadly related to each other:

- Pyrexia:
  A is diagnostic of appendicitis.
  B results from the effect of enzymes on the limbic system.
  C of unknown origin should be investigated with blood cultures.
  D results from pontine haemorrhage.

This style of question takes longer to read and answer, and if there are more than a few the time available for the examination may have to be extended.

There should be no double negatives. Single negatives should be avoided if possible (example 3, D). Try to include in the stem as many parts of the options as you can. For example, if the stem is "Arthritis: . . ." and all of the options start with "is a . . ." you could rewrite the stem as "Arthritis is a:" (see example 2, stem). Woolly stems such as "Concerning the obturator foramen:" are old fashioned and can usually be turned into crisper phrases.

Some words, such as "always", "never", and "only" are contentious or an obvious signpost to the correct answer and should not be used. Others, such as "often", "commonly", "rarely", "sometimes", "frequently", and "may", should be used very carefully. Items that use the verb "may" have a high chance of being correct (example 4, C and D). Exact percentages for incidence, prognosis, and so on should be avoided (example 3, E): they may vary widely from source to source. You could argue for using a percentage if the item is obviously wrong, such as:

- Atheroma:
  A   occurs in 1% of the adult population in the UK

but if it really is obvious, like this question, it is unlikely to be useful. Similarly, absolute values for biochemical and peak flow measurements, etc, should be avoided. It is better to say ". . . of three times the normal maximum concentration" so that differences in reference ranges can be taken into account.

The stem and option should lead logically. It is easy to write items that look adequate but are not proper English, as in example 4, A and E, or do not make sense, as in example 3, C, and:

- Pulmonary microemboli:
  A   impairs gas exchange
- Sickle cell anaemia:
  B   has two bands on electrophoresis

Tenses should be the same throughout. The present tense is the most usual. There should be no mutually exclusive or inclusive options, such as

- Serum α fetoprotein concentration is raised in:
  A   all malignant tumours.
  B   adenocarcinoma of pancreas.

If a word in a stem is used as a noun for most of the options, try not to let it become adjectival, as in example 3, C and:

- Bilirubin:
  A   is a breakdown product of myoglobin.
  B   concentration in the serum increases in cirrhosis.

Useful standard terms include "Characteristic features of X are seen in", "Recognised features of X include", and "X is typical of". Characteristic can be defined as a textbook feature without which the diagnosis may be in doubt, and recognised and typical as referring to established facts, but all three adjectives have essentially similar meanings.

15

The stem should not ask a question. The answer to "Which of the following . . ." is logically this one or that one rather than true or false. Another problem with this construction is that the verb used in the stem can suggest the answer. "Which of the following is . . ." means that only one of the options is correct; "which of the following are . . ." means that two or more are correct.

Stems with a double statement can be ambiguous. For example, does the stem "Causes of hyponatraemia and hyperkalaemia include" refer to causes of hyponatraemia and hyperkalaemia, occurring together, or to causes of hyponatraemia and of hyperkalaemia separately? Options with two parts similarly cause problems, because they may effectively ask two questons, as in example 3, B, and

- Gastric carcinoma:
  - A   characteristically occurs in patients with pernicious anaemia because of delay in gastric emptying

Having laboriously constructed your questions and found them to be faultlessly logical, crystal clear, and in impeccable English, you then come to the really hard part. It is essential that new questions are constructively criticised by as many people as possible. These should include your spouse, your children, your fellow examiners and, for undergraduate examinations, the examiners in other disciplines that are involved.

Timing and form-filling

On the day of the examination you will probably need to give the candidates some guidance on the timing of the exam and the way that they should fill in the answer sheets. For example, you may need to show them where to fill in their candidate number, centre number, and course code number. If the equipment that will be used to assess the computer sheets reacts only to pencil marks and not to ink the candidates should be warned of this.

Candidates may choose to write their answers in the first instance on the question paper and then transfer them to the computer marking sheet. They should be told that this must be done within the allotted time of the examination and that extra time to transfer answers will not be allowed. Even with this warning, and even when it is repeated near the end of the examination, it is surprising how often candidates fail to enter their answers on the computer sheet in the available time.

It is also worth emphasising that the question sheets as well as the answer sheets must be handed in at the end of the exam, if you don't want a large number of your questions to become public property. If the questions that you set are published, this is not a problem.

Marking schemes

The simplest marking system is to give one mark for each correct answer. This was done in the early days of multiple choice examinations but encouraged guessing, as there was no penalty for an incorrect answer. To overcome this, negative marking was introduced, in which an incorrect answer is penalised by deduction of a mark. While it is usual to penalise a candidate by one mark for each incorrect answer, in statistical terms this is too facile and is not an adequate deterrent to guessing; the penalty, depending on the number of questions asked, should be 1.4–1.8. A "don't know" answer does not lose the candidate a mark.

For each of the items of a multiple choice question, computer marking will generate a facility index and a discrimination index for the examination being assessed. These indices are based on the results of the candidates' answers in this exam; these values are therefore not absolute and apply only to the use of the question in this exam and not in any other. When used again in another examination the values of the indices may change. On the whole, though, there is good correlation between the responses of different candidates in different exams.

The facility index is the proportion of candidates answering the item correctly. Items with a high facility index ("easy" questions) can be acceptable if there are others with lower indices as part of the set of options, or if they are considered essential core knowledge. Easy questions can sometimes still discriminate well, and so the facility index shuld not be considered as a variable in isolation.

The discrimination index of an item measures how well it distinguishes between strong and weak candidates. This is done by comparing the answers given to the item by the candidates in the top 50% in the examination as a whole with those in the bottom 50%. The index shuld be a positive number: the cleverer candidates overall would be expected to do better than those who were struggling. If the discrimination index for an item is low, the item should be checked. When the index is negative (the poor students did better than the best students), the item is usually poorly constructed and the answer looked for by the computer may be wrong. As with the facility index, the discrimination index applies only to the examination for which it was calculated, and for a given item will change between exams.

The number of "don't knows" for each option is usually calculated, with the upper and lower half centiles of candidates being separated as above. The number of "don't knows" among the better candidates should be lower than among the poorer. If it is similar in both, there might be an ambiguity with the wording causing uncertainty.

Conversion of marks

Multiple choice examinations are usually marked by computer in a raw fashion and the results converted into predetermined bands to place the candidates into ranks of 1–5. Converting raw marks into bands can distort the relative values by compressing a range of marks into a single band. This can occasionally mean that a worthy candidate can fail even though he or she has achieved good raw marks and clearly knew the subject. Some examples of the problems with banding are illustrated in the box.

There can be a tendency to regard the band numbers as having quantity rather than simply rank, especially when marks for the multiple choice questions are considered in conjunction with marks for the practical, viva, and other parts of an exam.[5] For example, in the box a candidate who achieved 2 points from a raw score of 45 would not really be twice as clever as a candidate given 1 point with 35, or half as clever as a candidate given 4 points with 55.

Examination committees rarely make public the detailed results and assessment of their examinations. This is understandable, but as a consequence they are even more obliged to ensure that there is a proper outcome of the examination.

Assessment of multiple choice questions

All multiple choice questions should be reviewed by the examiners before each use to check that the questions are acceptable and the answers are correct. It is surprising how seldom in practice this is done. Ideas in medicine change with new discoveries, and out-of-date questions can be very confusing.

How banding can distort relative values

In an imaginary examination there are three unrelated subjects, each of which is initially marked out of 100. The marks in each subject are then converted to a close banding point system:

under 36	1
36–45	2
46–55	3
56–72	4
over 72	5

The pass mark for the whole exam is 9 banding points

- A reasonable candidate gets   46   46   46
  which is converted to   3   3   3
  and so reaches the pass mark of 9 from an actual score of 138.

- Another reasonable candidate gets   45   45   55
  which is converted to   2   2   3
  and so fails with only 7 points from an actual score of 145.

- A moderately clever candidate gets   56   56   73
  which is converted to   4   4   5
  and so receives 13 points from an actual score of 185.

- A very clever candidate gets   72   72   72
  which is converted to   4   4   4
  and so receives only 12 points from an actual score of 216.

Questions that consistently fail to discriminate between strong and weak candidates should be revised or excluded. Sometimes a question can appear to perform badly because the answer expected by the computer is wrong, and this sort of check can reveal the error before candidates suffer from it. Previous candidates in a multiple choice examination can provide useful feedback from the computer analysis of their responses in the exam: if there is more than one way of interpreting a point this will often become apparent.

This analysis can also show whether a bank of questions has been broken because the questions have become public, a problem especially of small banks. Simple changes to stems may be all that are needed to revive poor questions or to reconstruct the bank. When a multiple choice question is being run for the first time as part of an assessment, the results can be compared with previous candidates' performances in essay questions and vivas. New questions should not comprise more than about 30% of an exam, so that they can be compared with established questions on which analyses are available.

Public relations

A candidate's performance in a multiple choice examination should reflect his or her knowledge of medicine and not the ability to understand linguistic nuance. If use of English is to be tested, essay questions or vivas are a better way to do this. Sample multiple choice questions and brief instructions on how to deal with them should be available for candidates who are unaccustomed to this form of examination, so that results can be compared, for example, in different countries.

Verbal as well as performance-related feedback from the candidates about the questions can be very informative. Because of the extra time needed for them to write their criticisms, feedback is unlikely to be possible in qualifying examinations, when conditions must be strictly controlled, but in end-of-term examinations a blank sheet may be provided and an extra 10 minutes allowed for candidates to write their comments.

Conclusion

The multiple choice question paper has become established as a part of undergraduate and postgraduate medical examinations. Whether we like them or not we are obliged, as Anderson suggested, to "write good questions, evaluate them and appreciate their invaluable, if limited, place in assessment".[6] The first takes practice, the second is relatively easy, and the third may be difficult but should not be impossible.

1 Anderson J. *The multiple choice question in medicine.* London: Pitman Medical, 1976.
2 Slade P D, Dewey M E. Role of grammatical clues in multiple choice questions: an empirical study. *Medical Teacher* 1983; **5**: 146–8.
3 Lennox B. *Hints on the setting and evaluation of multiple choice questions of the one-from-five type.* Dundee: Association for the Study of Medical Education, 1974.
4 Vydareny K H, Blane C E, Calhoun J G. Guidelines for writing multiple choice questions in radiology. *Invest Radiol.* 1986; **21**: 871–6.
5 Ashby D, Baron D N. Harmonising multiple choice question marks with essay marks. *Med. Education* 1986; **20**: 321–3.
6 Anderson J. For multiple choice questions. *Medical Teacher* 1979; **1**: 37–42

Acknowledgement

I am grateful to Mr R C G Russell for his encouragement and permission to use some of the material in this chapter.

3 Take an examination paper

P R Fleming
Revised by John Anderson

Examinations in medicine today include a wide variety of written papers. The answers required range from lengthy essays to marks made by candidates on specially printed answer sheets to indicate their responses to multiple choice questions. I will first consider those questions that require candidates to convey their thoughts to the examiners in continuous prose—the "traditional" essay paper. I will then discuss those questions that seek answers in the form of brief notes—the short-answer question. After this I will consider questions that require answers of only a few lines, a phrase, a list of words or even a single word, best exemplified by the modified essay question and the patient management problem. Finally, I will discuss multiple choice questions.

Essay papers

The Preliminaries

The conventional long essay paper usually requires four to six questions to be answered, although some papers stipulate fewer and, rarely, some more than this. Depending on the number of questions that must be answered, the time available for each normally ranges from 30 to 45 minutes. Many essay papers are divided into sections and it is usual for candidates to be offered a degree of choice in selecting the questions they answer. It is essential that you read through the instructions printed on the paper so that you are in no doubt about what is wanted. It will sometimes be necessary, for instance, to write the answers to different questions in different booklets and you must always remember to write down the question number, both on the script and, when required to do so, on the cover of the booklet. Having read through the whole paper and noted whether any, or all, of the questions are compulsory, you should spend a few minutes planning your campaign. If choice is allowed, you should attempt to select the questions that you intend to answer. This requires careful thought, because occasionally questions that appear attractive at first sight become less so when you have started writing and find that your knowledge is less extensive than you originally thought. Whether or not you have to choose which questions to answer you must be certain, before you start to write, how much time you can afford to spend on each question. You must at all costs answer the right number of questions, as with most systems of marking it is difficult if not impossible to compensate for the omission of one question, particularly if it is a compulsory one, by submitting a brilliant answer of inappropriate length to another.

Planning your answer

Even when you have selected the questions you plan to answer —and remember that at this stage your selection may still be somewhat provisional—it is unwise to start writing immediately. Read the question you plan to begin with again, and make sure that you understand it. It is essential that you answer the question that is set and not the one that you would like to answer, as this may be an entirely different question. Study the wording of the question to determine precisely what it is that the examiners require. If you are asked to "give an account of the clinical manifestations of diabetic ketoacidosis" do not waste time discussing the biochemical features. It can usually be assumed, in a traditional long essay question, that "Discuss" and "Give an account of" really mean "Write all you know about". But this is not always the case. "Describe" is not quite the same as "Discuss"; the former requires a descriptive answer whereas the latter implies that deeper and more critical discussion is needed. "Compare and contrast" means exactly what it says. But you are still not ready to start writing! You must first plan, in rough form, the structure and content of your essay: what you intend to say. Sufficient time and thought must be given to this prior to writing the essay itself. For one thing, you may realise during this planning stage that you know less about the topic than you thought and, if a choice is allowed, you have time to select another question.

To reach an overview of the *structure* and *content* you need to decide the main aspects of the topic, the ideas and arguments, and the presentation of descriptions and evidence that will make up the body of your essay. Clarity in the relationship between ideas, descriptions, arguments, and evidence is one of the characteristics of a high quality essay. Relevance of content, cogency, and critical thinking are also essential attributes of a good essay, as well as being intellectual attributes essential to the practice of medicine. In determining the structure of your essay, planning by heading is one simple way to proceed. A possible outline structure for your plan would include:

- Introduction: brief comments on the subject of the essay or what you understand by it,
- Main body: several main ideas, each supported by evidence and argument when appropriate. Jot down headings and subheadings for this main section,
- Conclusion: it is helpful for you, and impresses the examiners, to draw things together and tie the essay up.

Writing your essay

No matter how comprehensive and accurate the content, several pages of closely written, continuous and unstructured prose without headings or paragraphs run the risk of losing the sympathy of the examiner, who might have over 100 scripts to mark. It is important that the examiner's immediate reaction to your essay should be favourable, so lay it out to reflect its structure. Paragraph it carefully into natural units and ensure that your main ideas stand out clearly. Use headings and subheadings, preferably underlined, to achieve this. Ask yourself how, if you were the examiner, you would react to what you have written and to the way you have set it out. By this stage, of course, it's probably too late to do anything about this, hence the essential need for careful preparation.

Style is important. Do not use long, tortuous sentences that are difficult to follow. Candidates are usually reminded of the importance of writing good English, but most examiners regard split infinitives and hanging participles with a reasonable degree of equanimity. This is not to say, however, that they will not be irritated by gross solecisms in style and frequent spelling errors.

Statements like "The patient should be PR'd for malena" are unlikely to improve your chances. Some examiners are touchy, too, about abbreviations, and you should be careful when using them. Such terms as BP, MSU and JVP are probably acceptable, but you should avoid "statements" like "XS dose of insulin → BG ↓ and LOC" as a substitute for "An excessively high dose of insulin causes hypoglycaemia, which may lead to coma". Remember also that some abbreviations (such as CT) mean entirely different things to different specialists.

Presentation is important; write legibly (nothing depresses examiners more than illegible scripts) and avoid unsightly crossings-out and corrections. Unless they are specifically prohibited, diagrams and figures—when relevant and carefully drawn—will usually enhance an essay, and flow charts and lists, when appropriately used, are also helpful. Above all, please write in prose and avoid presenting your answer in the form of short notes, unless you are expressly encouraged to do so.

Finally, I would repeat the importance of careful timing. An "essay" that consists of a single sentence and the frantic written plea "ran out of time" will gain you little credit with the examiner.

Short answer (short note) questions

A frequent style presents an initial instruction such as "Write brief notes on" or "Compare and contrast", followed by from three to six topics. Choice, if it exists at all, is much more limited than is the case with essay questions and is usually limited to selecting three out of four (or four out of five or six) of the topics that follow the stem. It is essential that you calculate how much time you have to write each answer ("user-friendly" examination papers will often tell you this). It is inevitable that only five to ten minutes can be allowed for the answer to each item, so it is possible only to set out the essential facts in your answer. Do not try to write a mini-essay; notes are usually sufficient. Tables, diagrams, figures, and lists are usually appropriate. Despite the limited time available, short answer questions test more than factual knowledge (for one thing, unlike multiple choice questions, you are not given any cues); they test discrimination— your ability to identify those points that are essential to the answer and to ignore what is irrelevant. Such questions will often be marked against model answers provided by the examiner, thus increasing their objectivity.

You should otherwise approach these questions in the same way as you do essay questions: read them carefully, make sure you understand them, and answer the question that has been asked. Do not answer fewer questions than are required, but remember also that, if there is a choice, you will not gain any credit for answering more than are necessary. Literary style and grammar are less important—these are, after all, short notes—but spelling is important and legibility even more so.

From time to time both essay and short answer questions are included in the same paper. The rules for these are as given above, but please make certain that you understand the type of question that you are answering. Note also that in such hybrid papers the short answer questions are often compulsory.

Very short answer questions

Increasingly, the format of some written examinations is such that candidates' answers consist of a few lines, a phrase, a series of words, or even a single word. Such papers include modified essay questions, patient management problems, and questions about projected material or printed photographs. In the first two cases the questions occur sequentially, separated by text that progressively develops a clinical problem or a series of problems. There are usually few difficulties, therefore, in composing the answers, but it is essential for you to pay attention to the instructions and to the precise wording of the questions. These are usually highly specific, and if you are asked, for example, for two possible explanations of a set of laboratory data, there is no point whatever in listing three. Equally, you must be specific in your answers; in interpreting a photomicrograph or a projected slide of a blood film the answer "Acute lymphoblastic leukaemia" for instance, will give you more marks than "Leukaemia". You will often have to prioritise your knowledge; for example, "Give the *three* most likely explanations for these findings"; "List the *four* most important investigations that are indicated"; and so on. *Read carefully, write carefully, and do exactly what you are told to do: no more and certainly no less.*

Multiple choice questions

Almost all of the multiple choice question (MCQ) papers included in undergraduate and postgraduate medical examinations in the UK use the multiple (or independent) true/false style of question, with an initial stem followed by (usually) five items. The stem taken with the item, or the items themselves (depending on the form of wording), make up a grammatical sentence or *statement*. Each item must be identified as either true or false; each is independent of all of the others. Candidates are usually, but not invariably, also given the opportunity to indicate "don't know". Each item has equal weighting, whether true or false. You will normally indicate your answers in these examinations by completing response sheets—drawing lines or filling in boxes—which are then machine-read by an optical mark reader (OMR). The output from the optical mark reader is processed by a computer that has been appropriately programmed.

The charge of unreality has often been levelled at multiple choice tests, and this point is well taken, particularly by those with considerable experience in constructing them. Nevertheless, the disadvantages are outweighed by the precision and reliability with which your factual knowledge may be assessed using this technique. Your sole aim in answering these questions should be to obtain as high a score as possible, and you are unlikely to achieve this by adopting a cautious approach and marking a large number of items as "don't know". The surest way to do well is to know the answers to all the questions, but strategy can also play an important—some would feel too important—part. In addition, it is essential for you to be able to communicate your knowledge accurately through the medium of the response sheets. For the clear-headed candidate who is familiar with the technique this should pose no problems, provided that you understand the form of the questions, follow the instructions given with great care, and read the questions carefully. Once more the golden rule is to answer the question that has been set, and not the question you *think* you read or would prefer to answer. You should therefore study both the stem and the items— consider the *statement* you have read—carefully. Then respond accordingly. Multiple choice questions are not designed to trick you, and in well conducted examinations ambiguous questions—whatever you might think—are rare. The examiners do *not* deliberately set questions that have hidden meanings or contain catches.

When you have read the question and are sure you understand it, you should indicate your answer by marking the response sheet boldly, correctly, and with great care. Take particular care not to place your mark in the wrong box. You will normally have the opportunity to erase an initial selection and to fill in an alternative.

In this situation make sure that your erasure is complete. In responding, regard each item as independent of every other item; each refers to a single quantum of knowledge. You should be aware of, but not pay too much attention to, grammatical "cues". In earlier days the permissive terms "may be" and "can be" had a tendency to be "true" in most cases, and absolute terms such as "always" and "never" were, almost invariably, false. However, experienced examiners are fully aware of these cues and will word questions accordingly. Be warned!

If, as is commonly the case, marks are deducted for wrong answers, you may be reluctant to attempt any questions other than those about which you feel absolutely certain. Such timidity usually means that you will do yourself less than justice. You must be prepared to use reasoning, deduction, and thought to score highly. Wild and random guessing is pointless, as you are as likely to lose marks as to gain them. However, just as action in clinical medicine is often necessary without complete information, so you must be prepared to "play your hunches" when answering multiple choice questions. Remember also that guesswork is not a good strategy when you are caring for patients. Do not be afraid to say "don't know" if this genuinely reflects your level of knowledge. But do not give in too easily. On the reasonable assumption that hunches are, on balance, more likely to be right than wrong, and provided that no more marks are deducted for an incorrect answer than are awarded for a correct one (the negative counter-mark is normally the same as the positive mark), this practice will almost certainly result in an improvement in your score. You will lose some marks by adopting this strategy, but if your judgment and reasoning are sound, you will gain more marks than you lose. Take chances, therefore, if you feel that they are reasonably safe and secure.

Do not count up the number of responses that you have made that you think you have got "right", calculate a score, and then (if you think your score is "safe"), mark "don't know" for all the remaining items. This is very dangerous because, firstly, you do not know what the pass-mark for the examination will be and, secondly, because some of the answers you are "certain" of will surely be wrong. Not only will you not gain those marks, therefore, but you will probably lose an equivalent number.

It is sometimes suggested that you should go quickly through the whole paper, marking down the answers you are "certain" of as you go, on the question paper itself if this is permitted, rather than slowly and steadily completing each question one by one. The former method has the advantage that it gets marks "into the bank", and avoids the risk that you may be left with several questions to answer, some of which you might know, when time is called. It also allows time for the review of difficult items that you missed out the first time round. On the whole I would recommend this "rapid" approach. As always, it is important to pace yourself throughout such a paper and, when the answers must be inserted on the response sheet, allow yourself sufficient time at the end of the examination for a careful inspection of the sheet for errors of transcription. However, repeated review of your answers may be counterproductive. Answers that you were originally confident were "absolutely correct" often look less and less convincing on repeated perusal. In this situation first thoughts are usually best, if you have read and understood the question properly.

In summary, therefore, you should:

- read the question carefully,
- make sure you understand it,
- accept it at face value,
- mark your selections clearly,
- mark in the right boxes,
- aim to score highly,
- reason out answers,
- avoid counting your responses and "sticking" when you think you are "safe,"
- *be bold and play your hunches.*

4 Organise a clinical examination

H N Cohen

Chance favours only the mind that is prepared.

Pasteur

The clinical examination is a trial not only for the candidates but also for the organiser, who has to ensure that candidates receive a fair assessment by providing a careful selection of patients and a calm environment for the examination. He or she must also ensure that all runs smoothly to allow the examiners to make unbiased judgments on the candidates. The combination of fractious examiners and flustered candidates, as a result of poor organisation, is bound to be detrimental to a candidate's performance.

Three to four months before the examination

Read carefully the examination regulations and any advice given to organisers from the examining body. Efficient organisation requires the cooperation and coordination of several individuals, so once the examination date is known, check your own availability and that of your colleagues, nurses, and secretary. You may need to reorganise clinics and holiday and study leave. Try to arrange for the examination to be held in a single ward, used solely for the purpose. Contact the nursing management to arrange for the provision of staff: smooth running on the day greatly depends on an efficient nursing team.

Two to three months before the examination

Prudent organisers will already have a bank of patients to refer to, but, if not, you must start selecting patients at this time. The examining body must tell you the number of candidates and sets of examiners who will be attending; once this is known, you must arrange schedules for the patients, who should not have to attend for more than four to five hours, that is, for either a morning or afternoon session. To ask a patient to attend for eight continuous hours is, I believe, reprehensible, and it is unfair to candidates, especially late in the afternoon in "long cases".

Long cases need not have any physical signs, but good histories (and historians) are required. The number of "short cases" per session can be approximately calculated from the following formula:

$$1.5 \times (\text{number of candidates in session}$$

$$+ \text{number of sets of examiners}).$$

One long case will generally be needed for each candidate. Any long cases with good physical signs should preferably be used early so that they can be used as short cases later in the session.

Short cases must have clear cut physical signs, as it is then easier to test a candidate. Poor candidates show their deficiencies more readily in their inability to recognise clear cut physical signs than in their inability to elicit equivocal abnormalities. At the very minimum, most medical clinical examinations require each candidate to examine cardiovascular, abdominal, neurological, and chest systems.

When you have decided the days and times that individual patients are required, you can send out a letter explaining the examination and suggesting time and date of attendance. Give the patient the opportunity to offer an alternative date in the reply slip and always send a stamped addressed envelope. Make it clear if lunch or transport is to be provided and ask whether these will be required. State the time the patient will be able to leave the examination and never underestimate this.

Keep an up-to-date list of patients' schedules so that you can reorganise if necessary to ensure a satisfactory number and spread of disease and physical signs. Make sure that the short cases are complete at an early stage. It is an advantage to have some long cases as inpatients at the time of the examination so that a prompt start can be achieved. I always send a second letter to the patients confirming the date and time that they have agreed to come.

Three weeks before the examination

Now comes the arduous task of writing summaries about the patients. These should be concise and consist of relevant information only. Do not use more than one side of A4 paper and usually considerably less. In short cases one or two lines will suffice, for example, "splenomegaly due to chronic lymphatic leukaemia". There is no need to elaborate; the examiners will assess the patients before the examination starts and make their own notes. The case notes of all long cases and any suitable radiographs or other investigations for long and short cases should be available.

Scripts of case summaries should be stapled together (long cases first), with a contents page at the front listing all patients, their diagnoses, and a number code that corresponds to bed numbers in the ward. There should also be a page showing the ward plan with beds clearly marked with their numbers. Always have a blank top sheet to prevent candidates seeing the contents page.

Check that nurses and porters know about the transfer of patients from ward to ward and the number of patients who will need lunch. If the regulations require it, obtain name badges and white coats for the examiners. Arrange to have well printed, clearly written numbers to put on to beds corresponding to the bed numbers on the ward plan. Earmark side rooms for each pair of examiners and a waiting room for candidates. Arrange with the catering staff for coffee, biscuits, and soft drinks to be available on each day of the examinations both for examiners and candidates. If possible, build into the time schedule a short break in mid-morning and mid-afternoon. Try to arrange a quiet, restful place in the hospital for lunch for the examiners and don't forget to buy some sherry. Finally, arrange for signposts to be put up around the hospital directing candidates to the appropriate ward, and alert porters and receptionists.

Examination day

Arrive at the hospital well before the examination starts. There will always be unexpected problems: the main road to the hospital may be blocked with snow; the coffee urn may have broken; the examination ward may have been taken over by decorators; your secretary may be off sick (the worst possible catastrophe); you may have forgotten to rearrange an outpatient clinic; or the key to the office containing the patients' scripts may be lost. There will be the inevitable last-minute cancellations by patients and a few "disappearing physical sign syndromes". Always have a few spare patients in the wards (especially with cardiovascular and abdominal signs) who can be substituted. A round of the main wards the day before the examination can be rewarding and will put your mind at rest.

Try to start the examination on time, as it is very difficult to pick up time if you begin late. When the examiners arrive, coffee and biscuits will promote a friendly start. Check the patients' physical signs yourself and then introduce them to the examiners; allow about half an hour for 12 short cases.

Have a plan showing when each candidate has to be with each set of examiners, and give the plan to all invigilators and to each examiner, so that there will be no confusion as to which examiners should be with which candidate and where. For example:

	1000–1100* Long cases	1120–1140 Short cases	1140–1200 Oral
Examiners		Candidate No	
A and B	215	216	217
C and D	216	217	215
E and F	217	215	216

* Allow for 15–20 minutes' questioning on the long case.

Conduct of the examination

Ensure that the relevant instruments are available on a trolley in a central area and that the ophthalmoscopes are working. Candidates will also require paper and clipboards; have a few pencils available. Patients used as long cases should produce a urine sample but must never be forced to do so. Try to keep the long cases separate from the short cases. Patients who require fundoscopy examination should be put in a darker area if possible. I generally dilate the pupils.

You will need one or more colleagues to help invigilate and to ensure accurate, synchronous timing and guiding of candidates and examiners. Registrars are a valuable asset for this and can help put candidates at their ease. They also find it a useful experience, especially if they can be paid a small honorarium. It is best to keep time from a wall clock in the ward that is clear for everyone to see. I usually give a half-time warning and a warning two minutes from the end to examiners, as well as a final warning by bell or alarm even if they say that they will time themselves so that I feel completely in control. Sometimes a little gentle bullying is necessary to ensure that examiners keep to their schedules. (I have never heard of an examiner complaining that lunch came too early.)

It is important that all patients are seen during the examination. Keep a mental tally during the session, and if a patient is not being used, inform the senior examiner and tactfully ask if the patient could be used when it is convenient.

When a candidate has finished, never succumb to the temptation to discuss the correct diagnoses even if the day has ended. This is unfair to previous candidates and will often result in concern rather than succour.

End of the examination

Collect all relevant paperwork that has to be forwarded to the examination body, and thank all the patients and staff who have helped. If the examiners have left any sherry, this may be a good time to offer some liquid resuscitation to the many staff who have helped in the invigilation.

Do not expect organisation of an examination to be a particularly gratifying experience, other than to give much personal satisfaction. You may be motivated by the proverb that "humility goes before honour" but you are more likely to feel, in Sir Walter Scott's words, "unwept, unhonoured and unsung".

5 Take a clinical examination

J F Stokes

So you are taking a clinical examination and are looking for some help to get you over this hurdle regarded by some as a half hour disaster session, and commonly painted in garish retrospective colours by those who have already tried to jump it. The first thing to do is to ignore the account of the man who said he failed because he missed the diagnosis of pseudopseudohypoparathyroidism in the short cases: it is more likely that he was unable to locate an obviously displaced trachea or found himself at a loss when invited to palpate for enlarged cervical lymph nodes. Clinical examinations are for testing your command of clinical skills, for finding out whether you can *do* things rather than simply remember, talk, and write about them. Don't expect to get by on bookwork; reciting 57 causes of haemolytic anaemia will not excuse your failure to feel an easily palpable spleen.

A live dimension

Though you may possibly have had some experience of showing what you can do with a dogfish, a cockroach, or a dead bacterium, a clinical examination introduces a new dimension, in that you are dealing with a live animal—one of your own species, and one that is quite capable of bringing some personal bias into your encounter. Fear of the unknown patient probably upsets some students as much as fear of the unknown examiner; this anxiety is accentuated by knowing that you will be spending some time alone with a patient, whereas you might normally talk to a *pair* of examiners, one discussing a problem with you, the other listening, which improves your chances of a fair appraisal.

Clearly the first step you must take is to ensure that you get lots of practice in talking to patients and in examining them physically; the more abnormal physical signs you have met before, and the wider the range of personalities you have had to contend with, the better. The latter is particularly important when it comes to taking a history, including a psychiatric history, for which you may need special training.

One of your problems may be the proper organisation of the time available to you, so as to be sure that you don't omit any important inquiry. You will, of course, take the blood pressure and test the urine; some people like to do these things early on so that they don't forget them in the race against the clock.

You must be absolutely confident about your ability to search for the apex beat of the heart, and have a clear plan in your mind as to what you are going to do when you can't find it—percuss the precordium, for instance, remembering that emphysema is commoner than dextrocardia. Be sure that you are comfortable with a knee hammer in your hand and that you appreciate that a niggling henpecking approach to the patella tendon may be as unlikely to provide a reflex as a smart blow on the anterior tubercle of the tibia. And have some idea of how an ophthalmoscope works. An earlier candidate, taking the view that the examination is competitive, may have left it for you with a + 20 dioptre lens in position and this will unsight you unless you know how to deal with it; remember that as soon as you lift your head you're going to be asked to describe what you saw, so check the instrument before you start—or carry your own. Though many doctors are arrogant in the way they hope to evaluate the retina in ordinary ward daylight, your examiners will have arranged for a pupil to be dilated if there is likely to be any difficulty (you'd better find out whether drops have been put in one eye—you might miss Adie's syndrome).

Don't be too hidebound by your training in a rigid framework of inquiry. Use an auriscope if you suspect the possibility of a cerebral abscess; examine the spine of a patient complaining of backache (this is sometimes overlooked), and the head of a patient with headache (rarely undertaken but capable of yielding impressive dividends in the shape of temporal arteritis or osteitis deformans).

It is more difficult to check on adequate history taking than on physical signs, but examiners recognise the overriding importance of taking a history in clinical practice and you will find that the assessment of this special skill will not be overlooked. Again, you should be flexible; you must be prepared to ask leading questions and to go to the heart of your patient's problem rather than play out time with a routine catechism. Some people may advise you to ask the patient three questions: "What's the matter with you?" "What treatment are you having?" and "What questions are the doctors asking about you?" That such an approach continues to be rewarding is due only to the fact that the examiners are not likely to be with you while you are taking a history (though they will watch you collecting your physical signs). Most examiners are aware of this problem and you will probably do better to take a history in the same way as you would if you were in the outpatient clinic rather than sitting an examination; this will at least protect you from such wrong footing as has occurred when the patient's answer to the first question was "psittacosis", interpreted as "silicosis".

Giving a good impression

As to dress and comportment, "neat but not gaudy" should be your watchword. It is at the clinical bedside test that examiners will try to decide what kind of a person you are and their judgment will have some influence on your final score even if it is not given formal weight. Don't be too upset by this random approach, which is already showing signs of being better organised in some parts of the world; in the meantime there are a number of points to which you can usefully pay some attention.

Wear whatever makes you feel comfortable—some men look excruciatingly uptight in an unaccustomed waistcoat. But don't appear more bedraggled than you can help and be sure that your hands and nails are clean; they will shortly be in contact with another human being who may well be spruced up for the occasion, and it is the least you can do. Give your patient identity; call her "Mrs Robinson" when you are asking her to take off her bra, not "granny", which she may not consider appropriate, nor "my dear", which may well be thought presumptuous on so short an acquaintance. It may be difficult for you, but try to relax; examiners get put out by signs of tension (sweating, overbreathing, and tremor all distract them from their job), and, although you may not find it easy to believe, they really welcome an opportunity for a quiet and uninhibited discussion with you.

If you're a man, you will have to give some thought to what tie you are going to wear; it should depend on how you feel when you get up on The Day—a bow, a recognisable club, or something anonymous —whatever is comfortable—but tuck it in if it is long, as it may exhaust the abdominal reflexes while you are auscultating the left chest. You also have to decide what to do with your hands, which are better out of your pockets.

If you're a woman, you have different problems; heavy rings may be uncomfortable for your patient when you palpate for axillary lymph nodes, long hair may flop over the anterior chest wall, swinging earrings get in the way. Your examiner may be an experienced man who is able to pick up a prophetic whiff of "Je Reviens", so watch your scent. If you are pregnant and it shows, you should be prepared either for an unnerving display of avuncular concern or for an unusually tough interrogation designed to convince the second examiner that no allowances are being made.

It is no longer so urgent as it used to be to discover the identity of your examiner. Pairs protect, and prophylactic action is taken by examining boards to avoid lethal combinations of examining genes. You will, of course, meet hawks and doves and the occasional peacock, woodpecker, cuckoo, or owl, but don't let this worry you; it will enlarge your experience and you may rest assured that, whatever their avian characteristics, the vast majority of them are trying to find out what you *do* know, not what you don't, recognising that an examination is no more than a milestone in a continuum of medical education.

Let me wish you good luck—you will still need a little bit of this.

6 Take an examination viva

N K Shinton

Preparation

The relative importance of the viva voce section of an examination varies from one examination to another. It may be the final assessment of the candidates and therefore of importance only to those with borderline results, or it may carry a proportion of marks. In some examinations it may be the method of deciding on distinction or honours. These are matters of immediate concern more to the examiner than to yourself so you should approach all viva voce examinations with the intention of conveying to the examiner the fullest possible extent of your knowledge and understanding of the subject to be discussed. The candidate's approach may be vital for success, but personalities vary from those who are overconfident and aggressive to the shy, timid people who find this part of the examination the greatest ordeal. Personality differences cannot be completely overcome, so it is better for you to behave normally and not to attempt to act a part, which, to your embarrassment, will probably be detected. A determined effort to be composed is always worthwhile but, in furtherance of this aim I wouldn't recommend tranquillisers, and hypnotics the night before can leave you overcome by sleep at a critical moment.

Opening

The moment of face-to-face contact between yourself and the examiner is very important, as first impressions can make the difference between a pleasant, comfortable interview and an unpleasant, irritating experience. For this reason, if you are neatly dressed you have an advantage over a candidate who is either slovenly or flamboyant. Likewise, your entrance into the examination room and the way you take the proffered chair can convey an impression of alertness or sloth.

The initial question is usually a general one to give you time to settle down and allow a rapport to develop. At this stage of the proceedings you must avoid repeating the question back to the examiner while you think of the appropriate answer, as this is a particularly irritating habit. Remember that the examiner will be listening to answers from numerous candidates within a comparatively short space of time. It is better to start talking about the subject in question and if possible continue until the examiner either indicates that he or she is satisfied or moves on to another question.

Answering

Testing your ability to communicate is the whole purpose of a viva voce examination. Always avoid vagueness or using words to take up time—no credit will accrue from this manoeuvre. Not infrequently the examiner hands across the table a photograph, specimen, or data relating to a patient for comment. It is a good principle initially to describe the exhibit and then say, if possible, what it represents. In the unfortunate circumstances that you do not understand the question, ask for it to be repeated, or simply say that you don't understand. If you really don't know anything about the subject, then say so because this fact will eventually be deduced and valuable time will have been lost.

You should appreciate that in the time allotted for your examination you must get across the maximum extent of your knowledge. Many candidates know the subject well but are unable to communicate their knowledge to others. If this is your personal problem, you should practice the art of communication or seek guidance from your tutor or supervisor prior to the viva voce examination. Should the exchange of views with the examiner lead you to the opinion that he or she has not appreciated your ability or knowledge, remember that there is almost always a second examiner listening who may well understand your answers. The purpose of having two or more examiners sitting together is to record as correct a mark as possible.

Distinction or honours vivas are, in practice, a battle of wits and knowledge between an above-average examinee and an examiner. The questions will certainly stretch the candidate's knowledge to the utmost, but for that reason may be quite enjoyable for all concerned. The process of determining your extent of knowledge may be long or short, so the length of the procedure is of little importance.

Closing

Whatever you consider the outcome of your viva, however disagreeable it may have seemed to you, always leave the room graciously. Even if you think that you have performed badly, try to leave a good impression, as it may not be so bad after all and in a borderline situation the final impression could be influential.

II ACADEMIA

7 Take a teaching ward round

John Rees

The traditional form of teaching in British medicine has been an apprenticeship and for many specialties the cornerstone of this teaching has been the ward round. This approach of basing teaching on close contact with patients is not typical of medical teaching in all countries, and in some British schools there has been a drift away from the bedside and into the lecture theatre and seminar room.

Medical educationalists have emphasised the importance of problem-based learning. The best place for problem-based learning is with a patient. Added to the clinical problem and its solution is the need to use skills of communication, history taking, and examination. The ability to record accurately and concisely the information in clinical notes can also be assessed.

What makes a good learning ward round? We all have memories from student days, many relating to charismatic, sometimes fearsome, consultants' ward rounds, but these memories often include the patients and their conditions. Recall of these patients presented on rounds is often far superior to memory of pages of textbooks and testifies to the effectiveness of those rounds.

The medical curriculum has become more and more crowded with the "essential facts" of each specialty. A course covering all possible options would have to be several years longer than at present. The General Medical Council recommends that the core of essential teaching in the curriculum be reduced, with choices of special study modules in the time freed. Bedside teaching depends on the patients available and it may be more difficult to ensure coverage of a core with this method. Lists of core topics and objectives for students and a diary to record their experience can help to make sure the appropriate areas are covered.

There is increasing pressure on teachers' time as well as on students' and there may be a temptation to combine business and teaching rounds. Resist this temptation. There is no harm in taking students on business rounds, particularly if they know about all the patients as they should, but don't be fooled into thinking that this can replace their teaching round. It is impossible to devote enough time and thought to teaching in the context of the business round.

There are four main elements to the teaching round: the ward, the patients, the students, and the teachers.

The ward

For many of us cuts in the numbers of beds and shared wards have removed the luxury of a personal ward and a devoted sister who would control the ward, maintain absolute silence during the teaching round and provide tea and sandwiches afterwards. Sanity is best maintained by arranging ward rounds clear of meal times and regular floor polishing sessions. Notes and x-ray films should be available and an accompanying nurse is an extra bonus, not least because it introduces students to a team approach to care.

All hospitals concerned in teaching should have a room available on each ward where the ward round can go to discuss the patients and the problems presented.

Patients

Some patients take great pride in displaying their clinical signs to anyone who shows the slightest interest, but such professional patients are in the minority. Others subject themselves to student ward rounds for a variety of reasons: realisation that students need to learn, obligation to the staff looking after them, and even a worry that refusal may prejudice their future care. Refusal to participate is unusual if patients are consulted beforehand, but they should be told what to expect and the time likely to be involved, and they should be given the opportunity to decline. They are more likely to agree if they have a student who sees them regularly and whom they identify as part of the team looking after them.

Patients need to be aware of what is happening in the round. They should be warned that discussion they may hear often applies to general principles and differential diagnoses and not necessarily to their particular case.

Patients to be seen on a ward round are, of course, chosen on the basis of availability. Few patients in hospital are incapable of generating an interesting ward round. There will always be aspects in the history, examination, investigations, social background, or treatment which are worth exploring. If not, then there is unlikely to be a good reason for their being in hospital at all.

Some discussion and examination will have to take place at the bedside, but, in general, it is best to move away from the patient to explore the importance of the findings and the management. A side room is best for this, out of earshot of other patients, who are less likely to understand the context of a ward round and quite likely to relate a garbled version of the story back to the patient—the ward bush telegraph works at impressive speed and range.

Shorter lengths of stay and more intensive investigation mean that some patients are kept very busy. A little preparation can avoid the problem of trailing from one recently occupied bed to another.

Students

Departments in many hospitals vie with each other to have the largest retinues available for their ward rounds. Anybody in a white coat will do and ability to understand English or medicine is not an essential qualification. These large white-coated armies have no place on teaching rounds. The optimal number depends a little on the experience of the students but is probably two to five. Larger numbers than this will be unable to see or elicit abnormal physical signs or to take an adequate part in discussion. One-to-one ward rounds can be intimidating for students, who miss the opportunity to learn from each other. There is no need for all students to hear a murmur or feel a mass on the round. Once the techniques have been demonstrated and one or two students convinced, others can return to see the signs for themselves later. Ward rounds should, however, be used to check on the ability of students to communicate effectively, elicit histories, and to examine.

If learning is really based on patients, then students should look after the inpatients on a firm and be able to present cases without notice. Some units do not run in this way and it is usually best to give prior warning, at least for the main case on the round. This allows the student and the teacher to prepare for the session. Most teachers have some topics that they would prefer not to discuss unrehearsed. It is possible to do so but it may limit the directions the round can take.

One of the best stimuli to student learning is the fear of examinations. The ward round has advantages here since it can mimic either finals short or long case format.

Teachers

The function of the teacher is not to give out information but to inspire the student to learn. When students have seen and discussed a problem on a ward round, they should be left feeling keen to go away and read further on the subject. This sort of patient-based or problem-based learning sticks much better in the mind because it has some immediacy and interest which reading page by page through a textbook or listening to a formal lecture can never have.

Few medical teachers have been taught formally how to teach and much of their technique comes from their own earlier experience of teachers. Courses on the approaches to small group teaching can be helpful although few deal with the structure of a ward round, where interaction with patients adds to the complexity. There are different approaches but the essential feature is enthusiasm on the part of the teacher. Most students will respond to such enthusiasm, and learning depends upon the response of the student; not passive transfer of information. Some teachers were enthusiastic in their use of ritual humiliation of students. Such rounds may occasionally be remembered with grudging affection 30 years later but it can take years for the scars on some students to heal and few teachers still carry on the tradition.

Teaching rounds are not lectures. If you want to give a lecture it is much more comfortable and efficient to move to a lecture theatre and talk to larger numbers. The ward round needs interaction—with the patient, and, most important, with the students. The round can be used to discuss points in the history and communication with the patient, to show physical signs, and to explore the techniques of diagnosis and management. Symptoms and signs in a textbook are just components of a list contributing to a diagnosis. In real patients they are individual experiences with their own unique features that can be further explored and interpreted. Few lecturers are gifted enough to bring their descriptions to life in the same way.

The round should be used to evaluate the students' diagnostic methods and cognitive processes. They should explore the processes they have used to come to their conclusions. As far as possible questions to the students should bring out this exploration, not to force students' thinking into a rigid format but to let them see the processes they are using and the alternatives available. This form of questioning and exploration is far more valuable than the provision of a list of the causes of clubbing or the familiar "guess what I am thinking of" approach. Facts and understanding will change during the students' careers, some even before they qualify, but the basic techniques of how to deal with these facts and fit them to patients' needs never change.

The number of patients to be seen on a ward round will vary. Students find long periods of standing on ward rounds nearly as tiring as operating theatres and they need to be conditioned. A reasonable length for a round is probably about an hour and a half, allowing time for hearing the history, demonstrating physical signs, and discussion. This allows time for reasonable discussion of one patient, or more if specific aspects are to be dealt with. Longer rounds are a physical as well as a mental strain.

The great importance of the ward round is that it deals with patients not diseases, it develops thinking processes, and it introduces the approach to patients that most doctors will follow for the rest of their working lives.

8 Keep up with the medical literature

Cindy Walker-Dilks

Keeping up to date with the medical literature is a never-ending task that begins as soon as one enters medical school. Medical information changes so rapidly and the publishing process takes so long that textbooks are often out of date before they are published. Keeping abreast of the latest medical advances requires access to the literature, selection of the right literature to read, and time devoted to the task consistently. How does a busy clinician have time to respond to this challenge? Fortunately for the medical profession, the medical literature is probably better organised than most other knowledge areas.[1] In addition, clinicians need know only a small fraction of the literature in detail because much of it is in the wrong area, or is redundant, invalid, or too preliminary.[2] This chapter will focus on methods for keeping up to date that consume the minimum of time, the sources to consult that give clinicians the most reliable information, and ways to store the information gathered in a usable form.

When faced with a specific clinical problem, the easiest and fastest answer is often obtained from a textbook on your shelf or a colleague down the hall. Textbooks are quickly out of date, however, and colleagues' memories can be faulty or biased.[3] Many more reliable sources are available to help you answer specific questions and keep up to date.

Database and journal sources

Medline is an excellent tool to use in the search for information. Produced by the United States National Library of Medicine

(NLM), it contains more than 7 million citations from 4000 journals, 60% of which contain abstracts, spans the years 1966 to the present, and is updated weekly. You can search it online directly from NLM, through other database vendors such as DIALOG and BRS, or search it on one of the CD-ROM products such as SilverPlatter. Although Medline indexes articles covering all aspects of health care, including animal studies and wet lab investigations, and various publication types, including editorial, opinion papers, and reviews, you can focus your search with the judicious use of subject headings and title or abstract words to retrieve a high proportion of citations to articles that are ready for clinical application, with a lower proportion of the redundant, invalid, too preliminary ones. Requesting studies that are randomised controlled trials in investigations of treatment or prevention, or that follow an inception cohort in studies of prognosis, will help reduce the amount of literature you will need to read to a more manageable and clinically applicable size. Selecting only this type of information reflects the recent shift in medical practice to "evidence-based medicine".[4]

A Medline feature that is particularly helpful for keeping up to date is the selective dissemination of information (SDI) file. It contains the most recent month of citations in Medline. Running a specific search in the SDI file once a month will keep you abreast of the latest articles in a particular topic area. You can run the search yourself, or arrange with a library or vendor such as NLM to run and send it to you.

Scanning the tables of contents of journals that offer the most useful articles to you is another method for keeping up to date, but you may not be near a medical library nor have the time to visit it regularly. Arranging to have the contents pages photocopied and sent to you or joining a journal circulation route with your colleagues so that certain journals are sent to you ensures that information regularly comes to you without requiring your active pursuit of it. Another option is to subscribe to a commercial updating service such as *Current Contents*. Published weekly by the Institute for Scientific Information, Philadelphia, Pennsylvania, it has two versions applicable to health care, *Clinical Medicine* and *Life Sciences*. A similar service is *Reference Update* from Research Systems, Inc., Carlsbad, California. These types of services are usually distributed in print, on diskette, or online, and contain the contents pages of journals from the health care field.

Abstract journals are publications that contain distillations of journal articles. *Journal Watch*, from the Massachusetts Medical Society, in Waltham, is issued twice a month and contains summaries of about 30 articles of relevance to all areas of medicine. *ACP Journal Club*, from the American College of Physicians, Philadelphia, is published bimonthly and contains about 25 critical summaries of articles of interest to internal medicine. The Oxford Database of Perinatal Trials contains summaries of randomised trials pertaining to pregnancy and perinatal medicine and will soon be extended to all areas of medicine through the Cochrane Collaboration.[5, 6]

Maintaining a filing system

Having identified sources that contain the most relevant and useful information, and methods to find that information quickly, you will want to retain and locate it easily. A personal filing system is a logical place to store your relevant literature, but it is useful only if it is maintained. Filing systems can be paper-based or computerised, alphabetical or numerical, and range from simple to complex.[7] The more complex a system is, the more work is required to maintain it. To find out what type of system is best for you, you need to ask yourself some questions. How much time do you have available each week for filing? How often will you use your system? What type of library access do you have? How many articles do you intend to file? How familiar are you with the material to be filed? Your answers to these questions will determine the level of complexity of your filing system and whether you need to computerise it. Material in a simple paper-based system can be held in a few filing cabinet drawers or boxes and filed by topic according to the chapter titles of an authoritative textbook or a controlled medical vocabulary such as Medical Subject Headings.[8] When the system grows to the point at which items are relevant to more than one file a decision needs to be made regarding cross-referencing, and the system is becoming more complex. A computerised filing system eliminates the need for cross-referencing and allows articles to have several access points. You can locate them by author, title, key word, or any other identifying information that you choose.

There are many personal computer filing software packages available.[9] Some packages have stored publication formats and citations styles, and allow for the assembly of a bibliography from a word-processed document. Most offer the capability of uploading citations from an online or CD-ROM search. Other features may include tailored formats for material other than journal articles, error and duplicate checking, and Boolean search capabilities (putting search terms together to broaden or narrow retrieval). Computer filing systems are powerful tools that can accommodate the filing requirements of your clinical research, administrative, and educational interests.

Conclusion

Keeping up to date with the medical literature is a life-long practice for clinicians and it is best to develop good information-seeking habits early. The curricula of many medical schools include training in literature searching, critical appraisal, and reprint filing, as medical students have discovered that they require these skills almost immediately. Knowing how to find information and being selective about what you read will help you keep up with the medical information explosion without the investment of excessive time or effort, and will maintain the level of professional competence that you and your patients demand.

1 Oldershaw J. Accessing the literature. *Br J Hosp Med* 1992; **47**: 433–7.
2 Haynes R B, Ramsden M F, McKibbon K A, *et al*. A review of medical education and medical informatics. *Acad Med* 1989; **64**: 207–12.
3 Covell D, Uman G, Manning P. Information needs of office practice: are they being met? *Ann Intern Med* 1985; **103**: 596–9.
4 Evidence-based Medicine Working Group. Evidence-based medicine: a new approach to teaching the practice of medicine. *JAMA* 1992; **268**: 2420–5.
5 Chalmers I, Hetherington J, Newdick M, *et al*. The Oxford database of perinatal trials: developing a register of published controlled trials. *Controlled Clin Trials* 1986; **7**: 306–24.
6 Chalmers I, Dickersin K, Chalmers T C. Getting to grips with Archie Cochrane's agenda [editorial]. *BMJ* 1992; **305**: 786–8.
7 Haynes R B, McKibbon K A, Fitzgerald D, *et al*. How to keep up with the medical literature (How to store and retrieve articles worth keeping). *Ann Intern Med* 1986; **105**: 978–84.
8 *Medical subject headings, annotated alphabetic list, 1994*. Bethesda, Maryland: National Library of Medicine, 1994.
9 Stigleman S. Bibliographic formatting software: an update. *Database* 1993; **16**: 24–37.

9 File reprints and references

Michael Marmot

Like most academics, I will shamelessly forget my ignorance and actually presume to lecture as if I knew something, but I have no such pretensions about filing references. I could hardly be counted an expert. I have not a single slide on the topic.

Why me? It cannot be because the former editor of the *BMJ* secretly visited my office and was impressed by the reference files. Why not ask an information technologist? If the editor wanted to know how to prepare breakfast, surely he would be better advised to approach Anton Mossiman than to ask me. I *do* know how to prepare breakfast in a way that suits me. But I would never be so arrogant as to suggest that it is *the* way to prepare breakfast.

A system that works for me is the approach I shall take in describing how to file references: not the Anton Mossiman approach to the supreme breakfast, but the approach of a humble breakfast eater who sometimes misses a breakfast, or finds that he has run out of oranges when his need is great. It is an occupational hazard of epidemiologists to be concerned with warnings of risks. Nevertheless, in this area, at least, I am much more comfortable with a list of don'ts than a list of dos. As everyone knows, to sculpt an elephant from a block of marble, you chip away all the bits that don't look like a bit of the elephant and what you are left with is an elephant. If you get rid of some of the bad practices, what you might be left with is a system that works for you. In case that is not enough I shall even describe two systems I have used: one off and one on the computer.

Why file references?

There are perhaps three main reasons why people accumulate reprints: photocopying takes less time than reading; the contents can be referred to at a later date; and a photocopy makes it easier to cite a reference when writing a paper.

The first is ignoble, and wasteful of both time and resources. Don't photocopy an article because you think it might be interesting and you haven't the time to read it now. There may be one or two people left working in health or higher education who still have access to all the secretarial or clerical help they feel they need, but they are not among my acquaintances. It is not a good use of your or a secretary's time to photocopy an article on the off-chance that you might have the time to read it later. Read it now, and then if you feel you must have it, obtain a copy.

It may be that the reprint-type services work well for some people— that is, those where you survey the contents pages of all known journals and fire off a shower of reprint requests every week. They don't work well for me. As with photocopying, it is easier to fire off a reprint request than to read an article. How many, I wonder, of the reprints dispatched in response to the requests that come thudding through the letter box actually get read?

But you are not that sort of person I hear you say. You do read first and then accumulate, but do you overdo it? It is very tempting to keep everything that may be of future interest, or that could be used in future teaching, research, or practice. But that is very expensive of time and storage space. Might it not be better to go back to the library occasionally than to accumulate vast quantities of references that are never again to be seen? Be selective. I know to my cost. When I decided to put my references on computer (more of that anon), it was so expensive (time) that I entered only about a third of them. In the subsequent six months I have had little need to access the dormant two thirds.

Why do you need a system?

Let us take what is, for me, a typical writing experience. You are writing a paper on alcohol and blood pressure. You need to remind yourself of how your results fit in with those of published papers. You pull out all the papers you have on the subject and you place your results in an appropriate context. Then comes the fun part.

You prepare the text and tables, and bask in a warm glow of achievement. The paper is finished, and you can now move on to preparing a lecture on depression and cancer. But it is not finished. There is the job of the references. You copy them off the papers you have, struggling with the spelling of foreign names and the opaque intricacies of the Vancouver system. As any editor will report, you do this appallingly badly. If you applied the same standard of accuracy to your data as you do to your references, your paper would, rightly, be bounced. In fact, it is possible that the reviewer of your manuscript may assume that you do apply the same sloppy standards to your data and bounce it anyway.

But then there are the references you don't have. You remember reading a paper by Mendeleev on vodka and blood pressure and you can neither find the paper nor remember the journal, nor for that matter whether it was by Mendeleev *et al*, or by *et al* and Mendeleev, or was it Stanislavsky? The infuriating thing is that you know that this very paper has been in your hands as you sat at this very desk and you can even picture the graphs of blood pressure showing a J-shaped relation with alcohol consumption. It then dawns on you that you pulled this paper out when you needed Mendeleev's address for a list you were compiling of European investigators interested in cooperative work, and if only you can remember where that folder is . . . . There are also, of course, the three papers you lent to, to . . . to . . .?

Even that hurdle is overcome. You send off the paper and now the work is finished. Regrettably, it is not. You are already deep into all the things you put off while you were finishing the paper, including the lecture on depression and cancer (which looks now like being a short lecture: it is depressing), and have not the time for anything as menial as refiling the reprints. That way madness lies. Next time you want to find those reprints, and experience shows that you tend to cite those same papers repeatedly, where will they be?

Entropy increases

The message of this story can be summarised by remembering the second law of thermodynamics: the universe tends to entropy. And this is nowhere more evident than with references. More specifically, remember a few don'ts:

(1) Don't delay in refiling reprints.

54

(2) Don't let reprints out for more than the time it takes a colleague to read them—they will drift.
(3) Don't construct a reference in Vancouver style more times than you need.
(4) Don't delay any longer in setting up a proper system.

We have one research fellow in the department with an IQ of 4000 who has read everything, forgotten nothing, and has copies strewn all over the floor, mingled with used squash gear, piles of computer printout, and goodness knows what. Most people going into his room can scarcely find the door, but in a race to find a reprint he always wins. Even he is now setting up a system that ordinary mortals would recognise as such. It is essential.

What type of system?

This can be split into two: (1) the system of filing the reprints; and (2) the filing of the references to them. The two are related.

By topic

The simplest system of filing reprints is to cluster them by topic. All your references to do with alcohol and blood pressure go into a file or box on that subject. This works if you have not too many reprints, or an infallible memory. The drawbacks of this simple system are obvious. When you come to prepare a paper on the public health response to the problems of alcohol, you have to search through the blood pressure file, the coronary heart disease file, the cancer file, mental illness, economics, motor vehicle accidents, plus the separate file you have on *BMJ* articles by Smith. Will you really remember which file yielded up which article, so that you can replace them in the appropriate one? This method might be appropriate for a topic that you might start to be interested in but you are not yet sure. For example, you throw everything you have read on the destruction of medical education by underfunding into one box, pending serious review one day (perhaps after you have been made redundant).

In alphabetical order

Most of us find the pressure to have a more systematic way somewhat irresistible. My choice was to file all reprints in alphabetical order by the first author's name. Others assign each reprint a

55

number as it comes in and file them in numerical order. Both systems should be supplemented by either a card or computer system of keeping references. The advantage, I find, of the alphabetical system of filing is that you can bypass your card system if need be and go straight to your files to find the paper by Mendeleev (provided he really was the first author) without first having to look up the paper's accession number.

References

My old system was cards. Two cards for each reprint: one filed by alphabetical order of first author, the other by topic. Yet, what if something belonged in two or more topics? I just had to remember. But at least I had two chances: either remember the author's name or the topic under which I had catalogued the card.

Computers

I was a reluctant convert to modern technology. I have a very elegant pencil and a yen for beautiful white paper, but in the end I shelled out a different type of yen for an electronic friend. One of the reasons was that I could no longer bear the pain of the references at the end of papers. The finding, the typing, the proof-reading (how do you spell Mendeleef?), or the changing from Vancouver style to some other form for that book chapter.

There are, no doubt, several reference systems and you will have to look elsewhere for a thorough review.[1] The one we purchased, Reference Manager (Research Information Systems, 1991 Village Park Way, Encenitas, California 9204, USA) works well, and scores quite highly in the *Which?* type comparisons.[1] You enter your references once on the Reference Manager system and **never** have to type that reference again. You can set up the system to produce your references in various styles, and when you enter the reference you also enter several key words. When searching for a reference, you can search on any of the authors, not only the first (you really can look for *et al* and Mendeleev), and on journal, key words, and title, or accession number.

The part that you really like to bore your friends with comes when writing the paper. In your unique database, *et al* and Mendeleev has the number 4006 because it was the 4006th reference that you entered in your Reference Manager file. In the text of your paper you cite the reference as {4006}. When you have finished the final final draft of your paper for the *BMJ*, the Reference Manager goes through the paper and replaces all the {4006}s.[2] It then constructs the reference list for you in *BMJ* format. Miraculous.

When I started using this, regrettably it cut my productivity by half. But that is my experience of each faltering step I have taken with the computer. When you get over the inevitable teething troubles that are almost always because you have done something stupid, the thing really works. I do now have my key references on the hard disk of my Toshiba Laptop and can actually keep editing anywhere. It keeps your mind off which part of the Boeing was last reported to have fallen off.

The other big advantage of a system like the Reference Manager is that you can lend references without parting with the reprints and having to worry about entropy. Anyone in the department can access my database to look up references and vice versa.

In the end that has to be the recommendation of this flawed, imperfect breakfast eater. One final word of warning. When you do decide to switch over to a computerised system, don't get caught halfway. The most frustrating position to be in is with a substantial slice of your references on the computer, but never the ones you want.

I had hoped to get to the end of this without any expertise at all, only bitter experience. In the end, my insecurity got the better of me and I sought the reassurance of an expert. John Eyers, assistant librarian at the London School of Hygiene and Tropical Medicine, agrees with the choice of Reference Manager, but warns that the system needs to be managed. If more than one person is inputting references, someone has to make sure that they are correctly input and a standard set of key words is used. He also supplied a useful reference.[2] But now is the time to set up your own limited database.

1 Wachtel R E. Personal bibliographic databases. *Science* 1987; 235: 1093–6.
2 Heeks R. *Personal bibliographic indexes and their computerisation.* London: Taylor Graham, 1986.

10 Choose and use a calculator

M A Mullee

In just over 20 years the calculator has been transformed from an expensive curiosity to a relatively cheap and sophisticated tool. Gone are the days when an affordable pocket calculator was considered advanced because it had a percentage (%) button! Today some calculators are programmable and have memories of up to 256 Kb, or more, some models accept optional RAM (random-access memory) cards, and some accept ROM (read-only memory) cards and can send and receive data via a personal computer. Calculators can now be used for the storage of information (such as addresses and telephone numbers), and some have extended dot matrix screens that can display graphics. Thus a great variety of calculators are now available, and before choosing one, the purchaser should ask:

1 What is it to be used for?
2 Will it do what is required?
3 Is it simple to use and is the manual clearly written?
4 Are its answers correct?

A brief description of the broad categories of calculators may help in choosing one appropriate to your needs.

General purpose calculators

As well as the basic functions of addition, subtraction, multiplication and division, hand-held general purpose calculators may also feature square root, percentage, sign change, and independent memory keys. In some cases the percentage key may allow the calculation of percentage increase, percentage decrease, one number as a percentage of another, and mark-up percentages.

The computation logic of these calculators should be checked before purchase. The arithmetic logic utilised by general purpose calculators may be different to that of scientific calculators. Thus $1 + 2 \times 3 = 9$ but $3 \times 2 + 1 = 7$ (operations performed in the order in which they are keyed) is the standard arithmetic logic used by the general purpose calculators of one manufacturer, which is different from the way their scientific calculators operate (see below). To avoid confusion, the symbol of the operator pressed may be displayed on the screen.

Many of these calculators employ solar panels to convert light to electricity, and some also have battery power, which takes over when the light is insufficient. Many battery powered calculators featue an automatic power off facility to avoid unnecessary battery wastage when the calculator is not in use.

In addition to the basic operator keys, desktop general purpose calculators may also feature additional memory, percentage, grand total, mark-up, item count, and constant function keys. These calculators may be solar powered, battery and/or mains operated, and some have a printer, with advanced models printing in colour.

Scientific calculators

Scientific calculators should employ an operator logic familiar to statisticians and computer programmers. This logic gives a predetermined priority to different operations; for example, it always performs division before addition, as in $1 + 4 \div 2 = 3$ and $4 \div 2 + 1 = 3$. Parentheses can be used to determine the precedence of operation, so that operations within parentheses are performed before those without parentheses: $(1 + 4) \div 2 = 2.5$.

The variety of functions performed by scientific calculators may include the calculation of logarithmic functions and statistical functions, such as summation, the sum of squares, the mean, and the number of data items entered. There may be two keys (σ_n and σ_{n-1}) for calculating the standard deviation. The formula for calculating a *sample* standard deviation is defined as

$$\sqrt{\frac{\Sigma (x - \bar{x})^2}{n - 1}}.$$

It is important to note that the divisor for the sample standard deviation is $n-1$, and therefore one always uses the σ_{n-1} key when calculating a sample standard deviation. Selecting the σ_n key effectively replaces $n-1$ with n and is used to compute the *population* standard deviation. As σ_{n-1} is the preferred estimate, the presence of this key (or its equivalent) on the calculator should be a prerequisite to purchase if the calculator is to be used extensively for statistics.

More advanced models may allow linear regression, quadratic regression, exponential regression, logarithmic regression, power regression, and inverse regression calculations. Some models have keys that generate random numbers, or compute permutations and combinations, which may be useful in the design of trials in medicine. They may also have a factorial key (n!, for example), which may be used in the computation of statistics such as Fisher's exact test.

The precision with which the calculator performs operations is very important if rounding of intermediate results is to be avoided. Calculators employ algorithms to perform operations such as computing a standard deviation. These algorithms may be written differently, depending upon the calculator model but if they are not particularly well written, they may produce inaccurate results. If possible, test the calculator to identify rounding problems. Storing intermediate results with the memory function will also help to avoid rounding problems.

Sometimes there are short cuts to performing statistical analysis. These are often described in medical statistics textbooks and should help when using a calculator. For example, Campbell and Machin[1] describe how to calculate the chi-squared statistic (χ^2) for a 2×2 contingency table. If the 2×2 contingency table is represented by the table:

		Variable 1		
		category 1	category 2	Total
Variable 2	category 1	**a**	**c**	**m**
	category 2	**b**	**d**	**n**
	Total	**r**	**s**	**N**

the short cut to calculating the chi-squared statistic is to use the following formula:

$$\chi^2 = \frac{N(ad - bc)^2}{mnrs}.$$

Some of the operations performed by the user may be quite complex and lengthy, and it is quite likely that mistakes will be made. Therefore, the manner in which the calculator handles the correction of mistakes (as well as the use of memory keys) is very important if the user is to avoid having to repeat the entire operation. This will vary from model to model, but some models allow cancellation of the last entry, or even deletion of the last digit entered.

Scientific calculators can be battery powered or solar powered with battery back-up to maintain memory contents and take over when light conditions are inadequate.

Programmable calculators

Programmable calculators allow the user to perform a calculation repeatedly by recording the keystrokes that are used to construct the calculation. The programmable calculator may have built-in formulae, covering mathematics and statistics as well as other fields. These formulae may be used as recorded or modified by the user and stored for future use. Programming devices may include conditional jumps, unconditional jumps, and count jumps. Graphics calculators are a type of programmable calculator that allows graphing of functions directly on to a larger graphics screen. The use of a moveable cursor may allow such things as intersection points to be identified. Graphing may also be built into the programming. The larger screen can display calculations, which can be edited. Some models also include a function menu system and a communication port that allows transfer of programs between machines. Programmable calculators may be battery and/or solar powered.

Other calculators

There are other types of calculator, which differ from those already described in a number of ways, not least because they possess a QWERTY keyboard, and a large display screen. Their memory capacity may be extended by additional RAM cards, so that it is possible to store modest amounts of data. They may also accept ROM cards containing programs such as a medical spell-check dictionary or spreadsheet (which may be data compatible with other spreadsheets such as Lotus 1-2-3). Advanced models allow communication between the calculator and the personal computer. These machines are generally battery powered.

Calculator or computer?

Despite developments in calculator technology, statistical analysis or laboratory calculations on all but relatively small data sets is probably best performed on a computer. It is for the user to decide, however, if (to retain portability) it would be more practical to purchase a portable computer—a notebook or laptop—for greater storage, diskette drives, processing speed, and the ability to use software packages not supplied by calculator manufacturers.

1 Campbell M J and Machin D. *Medical statistics: a commonsense approach.* 2nd ed. Chichester: John Wiley & Sons, 1993: 78–9.

11 Choose a personal computer

A J Asbury

Hardware and software

Start by ignoring the persuasive salespeople and colourful magazine advertisements and decide what you really want a computer to do for you. For example, do you just want to learn about computers or do you want one to help you write your MD thesis, manage the practice accounts, or do the calculations for your research project. Most people underspecify what they want. A common problem is that one buys a computer for the limited immediate purpose, and then discovers that it could have been used for other tasks had the initial specification been better, and a different, not necessarily more expensive, computer bought. In addition, decide whether you need a portable computer or a desktop model. In general, portables can do most of the functions of the desktop models, but the screen definition may be poorer and the data storage less.

The library is the next stop, where you should look at journals on basic computing, and particularly at the advertisements to see which computers and software packages (commercial prewritten computer programs) are available—and whether they will fit your funds. Most people buy computers to run specific packages, such as databases, statistics, administration, publishing, communication over telephone lines, accounting, games, or word processing. Look for review articles dealing with the software packages of interest and list the ones that you would like to use.

Now get some unbiased help to translate your requirements into a real computer description. It is particularly important with specialised applications to talk to somebody who really understands your application. If, for example, you are a general practitioner buying a computer for general practice, why not consult the Royal College of General Practitioners' computer experts, and, most important, visit a doctor who is actually using a computer in general practice. You might even decide that a computer is more trouble than it is worth. In addition, a local university computing department will usually provide unbiased advice and will welcome discussions with potential computer users.

Memory: hard and floppy disks

Check that the packages you want to use are compatible with the computer you propose to buy and that your computer has sufficient random access memory (RAM) to run the packages properly. RAM, the memory that holds only information while the computer is on, is able to manipulate information rapidly; if, however, there is insufficient RAM for a package, the program may run unacceptably slowly, or not at all. Most packages require at least four megabytes of RAM. Hard disks are usually permanently installed in computers and have very fast access times. You need data storage facilities to hold your software packages, data, and results in a form that the computer can easily use. Many modern computers provide a minimum of 80 megabytes of data storage on the hard disk, which is sufficient for most applications. You can also store data on floppy disks. Floppy disk storage is fast, reusable, portable, and inexpensive. A typical 5.25 inch disk might hold 1.2 megabytes of data, and a 3.5 inch disk will hold 1.44 megabytes of data; as a guide, a megabyte of disk space could hold 300 pages of single-spaced A4 text. If, however, you intend to store and manipulate images, one simple image can occupy 1 megabyte. A trap for the buyer is that there are several different systems of storing the information on floppy disk, and one should not assume that a disk of information written by one computer or program will necessarily be readable by another.

Printers

There are two main forms of printer. Laser printers are fast, usually quiet, often use standard cut A4 paper, but are fairly expensive to buy and to run. Dot matrix printers are noisier, sometimes faster than laser printers, can use fanfold or cut paper, and are cheaper to buy and run than laser printers, but the print quality is poorer. In recent years inkjet printers have improved, and they now produce fast, high resolution printing, in some cases with a quality similar to a laser printer. Laser printers and inkjet printers are reasonably quiet and will not disturb patients. All types of printer can print different typefaces in a range of sizes, and produce monochrome images (for example, graphs). Colour printers are available, but they are expensive both in capital costs and running costs.

Additional facilities

The mouse

The introduction of the mouse has made computers easier to use than ever before. A mouse is a small device attached to the computer whose movements on the desktop are sensed by the computer and translated into the movement of an arrow (cursor) on the computer screen. The arrow can be moved to point to text or picture (icon) items on the screen, and to initiate action. For example, the command to run a calculating package might be automatically given within the computer by the user simply pointing the arrow at a picture of a calculator representing that package, and pressing one of the buttons on the mouse.

Tape streamer

A tape streamer is a valuable add-on for a computer. It can store the contents of a hard disk on a tape cassette in 30 minutes, and the tape can be preserved against the disastrous day when the data on the hard disk gets corrupted. Data corruption doesn't happen frequently with modern computers, but when it does, it is time-consuming and highly inconvenient to re-enter all the damaged files. Restoration from the tape takes only 30 minutes.

Modem

Many manufacturers make modems, an add-on circuit that allows computers to communicate over telephone lines. Modems enable users to access major data collections, such as Medline, held on computers remote from them, and to collect data locally and transmit it over the telephone lines to a central computer for analysis.

CD-ROM player

A CD-ROM (compact disc-read-only memory) is an inexpensive method of storing large amounts of data—1000 megabytes. Some medical textbooks are already available as CD-ROMs, as are some encyclopedias and dictionaries. The CD-ROM player allows the user to read the CD just as one would read a book, but with the powerful additional facility of being able to search the whole CD very quickly.

Image handling equipment

A scanner can be connected to a computer, and is able to turn an image on paper into an image that can be displayed and manipulated on the computer screen. Such images can then be included in printed documents to give a very professional presentation. Images can also be generated on computers—for example, graphs produced by a statistics package; printed on a laser printer they are suitable for reproduction in journals. Images can also be passed directly from the computer to slide-making equipment, which can present the dilatory research worker with slides in an hour. All image handling equipment is expensive, and the images need considerable hard-disk storage. If image handling is anticipated, there are additional compatibility considerations, and specialist advice is necessary before buying.

Final decisions

Having defined one's requirements, the field should have narrowed considerably. Scan the relevant journals again for reviews dealing with your shortlisted computers and software; if necessary take the reviews and discuss them with your long-suffering expert. It is worth finding out where your favoured few stand in the market, and asking questions such as: Is the market price due to fall soon? Is the computer due to be superseded by another model? Are parts likely to be available? Is the computer reliable? Is the documentation good? Is there a local user group nearby? What maintenance contracts are available? Some companies run a phone-in help service for their users, and though you obviously pay for such convenience, it, like good documentation, can save you time.

When you know what you want, seek the most favourable deal.

Many manufacturers advertise the price of the "bare system" without cables or documentation, so check precisely what you get for your money. You may be able to negotiate a reduced price by buying all your requirements through one dealer, but ensure that this does not compromise your guarantee.

It is often convenient to buy your chosen computer through a magazine advertisement, but there can be disadvantages. Suppose that you send your money and the goods are not delivered in a reasonable time. The company may be holding on to your money "until stocks arrive", which might take some time. It could be that your requirements were not really so specific after all, and that your second choice would be equally suitable—and readily available down the road. If you are dealing at long distance, you cannot easily apply pressure on the supplier. The same reasoning applies to getting your equipment serviced. Servicing and repairs always take longer if you have to send the apparatus away by post, compared with visiting your local dealer. If you do send your computer away for repair, don't forget to insure it.

Some companies helpfully install and check your additional equipment (for example a CD-ROM player) before dispatch. If this is the case, make sure you know exactly how this has been done, that you have the full manuals and disks, and that the guarantee on the additional equipment is secure. Similarly, if your purchased software packages are installed, make sure you have the original manufacturer's disks; they may be needed to prove ownership of the software or to claim an upgrade at a reduced price.

Now reach for your cheque-book.

12 Use a word processor

Nicholas Lee

Word processing is one of the first tasks that most users wish to undertake on their computer; indeed, it is often the principal reason for buying a computer. Word processing covers a wide range of programs from the simplest text editor to powerful desk top publishing. Before deciding which word processing program to use or which computer to buy, decide what tasks you wish to undertake. Simple letters or reports can easily be done on a text-based word processor, of which WordPerfect for the DOS operating system is the one most widely used in hospitals and general businesses. Here the words appear as plain text on the screen and bear little resemblance to the final printed form. They are very much geared to fast keyboard operators, having their own combination of key strokes to manipulate and format the words. As with any software, do not expect to start the program and be an expert overnight. WordPerfect has been developed over an extensive number of years and has a huge variety of features. To learn how to use it to its fullest does take some time, but it is worthwhile. Once you have invested a significant amount of time in learning a particular word processing program there is usually a great reluctance to change to another because of the new learning curve.

For anything more complicated than a simple letter or report, a WYSIWYG (What You See Is What You Get) word processor is better. With these you will see on the screen exactly how the printed page will look and the effect of any alterations can be immediately appreciated before the page is printed. In addition, major programs such as WordPerfect, AmiPro, and Word have expanded the capabilities of word processing to include a range of other facilities. The great advantage of a text-based DOS program is that it runs very quickly on the most basic computer. The more powerful WYSIWYG word processors move away from the keyboard somewhat, utilising a pointing device, the mouse, to effect functions or to highlight and move text and pictures. Because these programs operate in the more demanding graphical computer environments a faster computer is required to run them with any speed.

WordPerfect is the commonest word processing program and is very widely used in hospitals. The great advantage in using the same software that your secretary and colleagues use is that you can easily transfer documents from one computer to another. Having said this, most word processors do allow you to both export and import text from different programs, though this is not always 100% successful.

Basic functions and features

Editing

The advantages of a word processor over a typewriter are that it is easy to change what you have written before it is printed; you can store your work so that you may return to it on another day and change or add to it as many times as you like; pieces of text may be easily moved around, copied, replicated or transferred into another document; frequently used phrases or paragraphs can be saved and incorporated into documents without having to retype them; and you can have several documents open on the screen at the same time so that they can be edited together.

Writing tools

Spell checkers

There is a wide range of writing tools available both within the word processor program and separately. The most useful one is the spellchecker, which will compare your words against a dictionary of the most commonly used words. Only a few medical words will be included, but you can add words to create your own dictionary. Obviously you need to ensure that any words you add are spelt correctly. Alternatively, those who use WordPerfect can add *Stedman's Medical Dictionary*, which contains 165,000 correctly spelt medical terms and generic drug names, to the spellchecker. When the spellchecker identifies a word you have used that is not in its dictionary it will assume that you have misspelt one that is, and it will list words similar in spelling, from which you can select the correct one and with one keystroke replace the original word.

Grammar checkers

While spell checkers will detect misspelt words, they will not detect incorrectly used words such as "to" instead of "too" or "two" or the absence of a full stop. Grammar checkers will detect such grammatical errors and suggest alerations.

Thesaurus

Lost for words? Then using the word processor's thesaurus may help you find the one you need. Other writing tools include templates for standard letters and a dictionary of quotes for that all-important phrase. If your computer has a compact disc (CD) facility, you will find that an increasing number of reference books, including a 29-volume encyclopaedia and the complete *Oxford English Dictionary*, with 55 million words, are available on CD-ROM (read-only memory).

Macros

A great deal of effort has gone into developing features to make writing documents as quick and as easy as possible. A macro programming language allows you to add your own short cuts by replacing a series of keystrokes or commands with just one keystroke, so greatly speeding up performing various functions. For example, a simple macro of the key combination "Alt-P" could be used to print the current document without having to run through the print menu. Complex macros can be devised for creating discharge summaries. In this way you can customise your keyboard so that your most frequent lengthy tasks can be operated from just a single press of a key combination.

Styling type

Different typefaces and styles were once the domain of the professional publisher, but now these are available on even the humblest word processor. There are thousands of different typefaces, or fonts, available. The commonest ones are Times Roman and the various forms of sans serif faces. These are all proportional fonts, which adjust the space allowed for each letter depending on

8 point Times Roman

12 point is the most commonly used size

24 point

Bold 12 point

Italic 12 point

Shadow 12 Point

Superscript and Subscript

SMALL CAPITALS VS NORMAL CAPITALS

Redline type

~~Strikeout~~

Outline font

Fine, Small, Large, Very large, Extra large

Colour Printers allow colour printing

White on black background

Special characters: é ç ñ † ⅝ ½ α Σ ₰

Fig 1 Examples of attributes that may be applied to a particular font

whether it is a thin letter like "i" or a wide letter like "m". This makes the text easier to read than the monospaced type styles in which each letter occupies the same amount of space. In a particular typeface, such as Times Roman in fig 1, there are a number of additional attributes that may be altered, including the size, which is measured in points; the position on, above or below the line; the weight, which might be light, medium, or bold; and the style, such as italic, outline, or shadow.

Tables

Tables divide the page into separate boxes, allowing columns or rows of text or numbers to be aligned. Not only is this useful for producing a results table for publication, but with the numerical spreadsheet capabilities in many integrated packages simple summing of columns and complicated mathematical calculations can be performed within the tables. Data can also be imported from, and exported to other spreadsheets or database programs.

71

Stationery

With a quality printer there is no need to have customised stationery printed because you can create it on your computer. This gives you great flexibility in altering letterheads and memo and report forms at any time. There are also letter templates available for many different kinds of business and personal letters, helping you use the correct form in replying.

Mail merge

This is a very useful way of personalising a circular letter to a group of people. To perform a mail merge you need a letter template with codes for the personalised details and a second file with all the personalised details for each letter. The computer merges these two files to create the personalised letters, saving the amount of time it would have taken to type each letter individually.

Forms

Printed forms, particularly the multipage self-carbonating ones, cannot be put through a modern printer. Since most modern forms will have been created on a computer, it is often possible to re-create them on your own computer. This is particularly useful with forms that you use regularly, such as police statements, abstract forms and claim forms. WordPerfect Informs is one example of a computer equivalent of a paper form. The form is generated on the computer, and then can be printed out or distributed by electronic mail (e-mail). If the form is sent by e-mail the recipient can fill it in on the computer, give it an electronic signature and apply a TamperSeal before sending it back.

Saving

One of the great advantages of the computer is its ability to store and later retrieve your documents. You can store thousands of documents on a computer, though finding a specific one can be difficult unless you label your files very precisely. Programs like WordPerfect's Quickfinder are very helpful. They create an index of every word in the documents you have saved and can search it to locate a single word or a combination of words in a specific document, which can then be retrieved. Important documents should be saved not only on the computer's hard disk but also on a floppy disk as a back up in case the hard disk fails and all the stored data is wiped off, or the computer is stolen.

Security

If the computer is stolen, all your confidential letters and patient notes will be immediately accessible to anyone switching on the machine. Most computers have a protection system built that requests a password as soon as you switch on the machine, and you should ensure that this is activated. This will stop amateur unauthorised attempts to access your files. Many computers also allow individual files to be password-protected, giving a further level of protection. More elaborate systems encrypt the data for those requiring a higher level of security. It may well be necessary for you to register under the Data Protection Act if you are storing names, addresses and other personal information on your computer.

Additional facilities

The fax

In our society high speed communication is now becoming the norm. We can send letters or documents to other people within a few minutes by fax, which makes the post seem very slow. There are two types of fax machines.

Internal fax modem

This either fits inside the computer or plugs into the serial port at the back of the computer and then into a phone socket. Programs like WordPerfect for DOS and any Windows-based package allow you to fax directly from the word processor without having to print the page. This system is better than the stand-alone fax for sending faxes since they are of near-letter quality, but it is not so convenient for receiving faxes.

Stand-alone fax machine

This is ideal for receiving faxes, being left on 24 hours a day and giving a hard copy. It allows you to send diagrams, photos, handwritten notes and other documents not created on the computer. But because the page has to be scanned, the quality of the received fax is not as high as one generated and sent from an internal fax modem.

Scanners

Adding pictures, arrows, boxes or diagrams to handouts or reports will greatly enhance their impact. These can be generated by the drawing programs included in many word processors or copied from other documents using a scanner. The scanner can be either hand-held or a large flatbed. A scanner using Optical Character Recognition (OCR) software can "read" typed, printed, and even handwritten text directly into the computer, saving the time and expense of retyping. For even a few pages this can save time, though it is easier to type a few paragraphs afresh.

Speech recognition

For those that dream of sitting back in their armchair and speaking into their computer, read on. The way we put information into computers has been changing and improving over the years. We have had ticker tape, punch cards, keyboard, mice, pull down menus and it is but a natural evolution to expect to dictate directly to the computer. Voice recognition by the computer has now been achieved and it is possible to dictate text directly into a computer at up to 125 words a minute, which is a fast speed for a typist. In addition, you can use voice to contol the computer and edit your text. In time using a keyboard will seem as outdated as punch cards do today.

Help

It takes time and practice to learn how to use a word processor, and everyone has problems with their computer occasionally. When you have a problem, take yourself slowly through the program and if you get stuck there is plenty of advice on hand (box).

Conclusion

The word processor has grown from being just an improved typewriter to being really a writer's assistant, doing everything to make preparing documents as easy as possible. It may seem a daunting tool to master at first, and this chapter has only touched on the features and functions available to you, but take the time and trouble to learn and it will become second nature to use.

Sources of help

Program manual	The book that comes with your software is, unfortunately, often not very helpful, but try it first.
Third party books	These are written by users for users, and are more readable than the manuals.
Help desks	All software companies have help desks that can be a useful source of help over the telephone or by fax.
IT help desks	Many hospitals have their own IT help desks.
Colleagues	Your problem will not be unique, so talk to your colleagues.
User groups	Many software programs have user groups.
On-line support	This is available via your modem (a device that links your computer to another by telephone).
Courses	The quickest way to learn a new technique is to attend a course.

Useful sources

Word processing software
AmiPro: Lotus software's mainstream work
processing package   01784-455445
CA-Textor: Computer Associates DOS and
Windows word processor   01753-577733
ClarisWorks: integrated software for Apple
Mackintosh users, now available for the PC   0181-756-0101
PC-Write: one of the best Shareware packages   *see* Shareware
Fine Words: budget word processing program   01453-753955
Starwriter: budget graphical (WYSIWYG) word
processing program   01533-626999
The Universal Word: a graphical word processor
that handles foreign languages such as Arabic and
Greek   01344-303800
Word: Microsoft feature-laden word processing
package   01734-270000
WordPerfect: most popular word processing
program, widely used in hospitals   0800-177277

Wordstar: one of the oldest programs on the market	0181-789-2000

Utilities

Adobe: wide range of fonts	0800-232223
Bitstream: wide range of fonts	01242-227377
Fonts: wide range available from Monotype; *see also* Shareware	01737-765959
Grammatik: grammar checker	0800-177277
IBM Personal Dictation System: allows you to dictate directly into the computer	01329-242728
IBM Translation Manager: assists in translating documents	01329-242728
Oxford English Dictionary: concise or complete on CD-ROM	01865-267979
PC-Index: automatically indexes your document	*see* Shareware
Stedman's Medical Dictionary: adds medical terminology to WordPerfect's dictionary; British and American versions available	0171-385-2357
Wordstar writing accessories: Correct Letters, Correct Quotes, Correct Grammar, Encyclopedia	0181-789-2000

Organisations

Many companies give medical and educational discounts.

CompuServe: wealth of information and help available on your computer via a modem	0800-289458
Data Protection Register, Springafield House, Water Lane, Wilmslow, Cheshire SK9 5AX	01625-535711
Shareware products: can be bought from Shareware libraries such as Public Domain and Software library	01892-663298
WordPerfect User Group of the UK: offers meetings, newletter, help and advice for WordPerfect users	01277-212545

13 Present numerical results

M J Campbell

When you cannot measure it, when you cannot express it in numbers, you have scarcely, in your thoughts, advanced to the stage of Science, whatever the matter may be.

William Thompson, Lord Kelvin

Data summary

The results of an investigation, which may have taken years of work, will be summarised in a few numbers that can be communicated in a brief conversation. It is important that these numbers are well chosen to encapsulate the main results of the investigation without misleading the reader. A common problem is how much detail to give. Should all the measurements be given? Usually some measure of location, such as a mean, is given, or the mean with some measure of variation, such as a standard deviation. It is worth recalling that it is only for Normally distributed variables—that is, variables that have a characteristic bell-shaped distribution—that the mean and standard deviation summarise all the essential information about the variable. For variables that are not Normally distributed it can be useful to give other statistics, such as the median, together with or instead of the mean, and perhaps the interquartile range instead of the standard deviation. The age of a set of subjects is unlikely to be Normally distributed, so that a range is more useful than the standard deviation.

One should always bear in mind the measurement accuracy of the data. It makes little sense to quote a summary statistic with five decimal places when the original data are rounded to the nearest unit, even if the computer printout presents it as such. Since summary statistics are estimated with more accuracy than the original data, one or two significant digits beyond the accuracy of the original data would suffice. For example, if height were measured to the nearest centimetre, that is, to three significant figures, then the mean could be given to four or five significant figures. Nominal or categorical data, such as sex or racial group, are summarised as percentages, but the numerator and denominator must be given as well. For total group sizes of less than 100 percentages could be rounded to the nearest whole number, for example "7% (2/30) patients subsequently died".

It is important to distinguish between the two types of data summary: *descriptive*, to show the distribution of the variables, and *comparative*, to show the main outcome of a study. In the former, in a clinical trial, for example, we would like to describe the trial participants by treatment group in a reasonable amount of detail, since trial participants are not a random sample of the general population and the reader would like to know who they are. At the start of a report one should include demographic data, clinical characteristics, and initial severity of the condition. Numerically discrete data, such as number of attacks of asthma a week, can be summarised by a mean, but it is often also worth quoting the median, since the distribution is likely to be skewed. The standard deviation is unlikely to be useful in this latter case, and variability could be summarised by the range or interquartile range.

In contrast, when reporting the results of a comparative study, it is the result of the *comparison*, for example, the difference in means, that is important, not the results from each individual treatment. The statistic associated with the variability of estimates (as opposed to individuals) is the standard error. More useful, but usually derived from the standard error, is the confidence interval for the differences in main effects, which should be quoted, since it measures the precision of the estimate. For example, in a study to compare PERF in schoolchildren with asthma who regularly use an inhaled steroid and those who use a bronchodilator, it is the *difference* in mean PEFR between the groups that is important, not the mean PEFR for each group. Details on calculating confidence intervals are available,[1,2] and so are confidence intervals associated with non-parametric tests, such as the Mann-Whitney U test.

In a report of a clinical trial one often sees an initial table describing the baseline features of the subjects, such as their age, sex, and disease severity, by treatment group. The purpose of this table is descriptive, to describe the patients in the trial. As such the appropriate measure of variability is one relating to the population, such as a standard deviation or a range, and not one relating to an estimate, such as a standard error or a confidence interval. A useful mnemonic is that standard deviation has a "d" for description, standard error has an "e" for estimation.

Units and symbols

All quantitative summaries should have the unit of measurement attached. Whatever units were used to carry out the work reported upon should be translated into SI units for publication. A few minor points are that the international symbols for hour and seconds are h and s, not hr and sec; no symbol has a plural form—10 mg, for example, does not have an s, and the ± symbol should be avoided, and (SD) or (SE), as appropriate, given instead.

Tables

Most results from an investigation will be summarised in a table. Tables, rather than figures, are the best means of conveying complex information accurately. A table should be arranged in a logical order that allows a reader to make comparisons or draw inferences easily. It is usually easier to make comparisons horizontally so, for example, results from a two-group experiment would have the variables listed vertically, and the summaries from each group adjacent to one another. In a scientific paper the author should always give the table a heading, and explain the contents more fully in the text. The table itself should have three horizontal and no vertical lines. The first and third horizontal lines mark the top and bottom of the table, and the second separates the heading within the table from the columns below them. The number of observations should be stated for each result in a table. Tables in which the rows do not have a natural order, for example, giving information on individual patients, are easier to read if the rows are ordered according to the level of one of the variables presented.

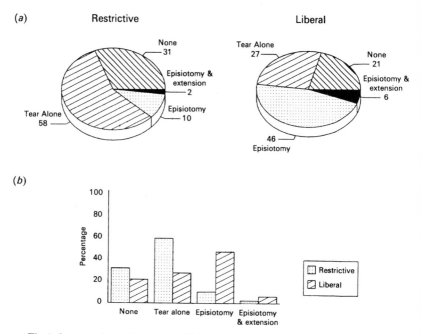

Fig 1 A comparison of outcome of labour under two policies: (*a*) pie charts and (*b*) bar chart.

Figures

There are two main reasons for displaying data in figures rather than tabulating them. Firstly, the human eye is better at detecting patterns in pictures rather than in numbers, and so the qualitative results of a study are conveyed rapidly to the reader. Secondly, a figure can convey a great deal more information about a study for a given amount of space than a series of numbers.

A useful reference is Tufte, who suggests that, within reason, one should maximise the ratio of the amount of information to the amount of ink.[3] Discrete data are summarised as percentages, and pie charts are often used to display them. While pie charts are useful in glossy publications such as annual reports, they are of little use in scientific work when comparisons have to be made, since the human eye is not very good at measuring angles. Consider the results from outcome of pregancy given in fig 1a.[4] Using the pie charts it is difficult to compare the outcome for restrictive and liberal

80

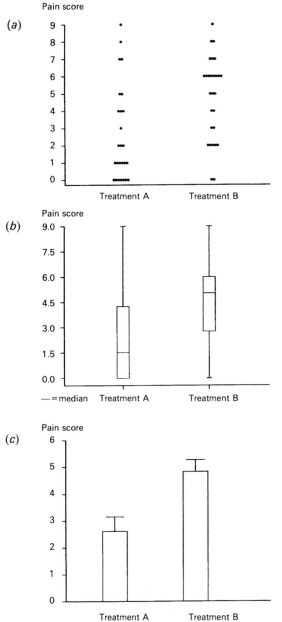

Fig 2 (a) Dot plots comparing pain scores under two treatments; (b) box whisker plot showing same data; (c) "dynamite plunger", mean and standard error showing same data. This plot is not recommended.

81

management of labour, whereas comparisons are easily made with the bar chart in fig 1b.

For quantitative data, figures that show individual data points are to be encouraged, since they contain a large amount of information relative to the amount of space and they enable readers to obtain the approximate raw data. Dot-plots can show distributions of continuous data. If the sample size is large (say, more than 50) and a dot-plot is too crowded, then box-whisker plots[2] are useful. Figures 2a and 2b illustrate the use of dot-plots and box-whisker plots to compare pain scores (on a scale 0 to 10) in two treatment groups. Since the sample size is small the dot-plot conveys all the information available in the data quite economically. Definitions of box-whisker plots vary, but in a simple definition the points are, in ascending order, the minimum value, the first quartile, the median, the third quartile and the maximum, and these are often sufficient to convey the main points about the data. An elaboration shows possible outliers by defining the whiskers to have a length as a proportion of the interquartile range (commonly 1.5 times). Points outside this range are displayed as dots. In this way odd extreme points do not distort the impression of the data. Contrast these displays with the bar chart showing a mean value, with an "error bar" (sometimes referred to as "a dynamite plunger plot"), in fig. 2c. "Error bars" are not universally defined, but are usually the standard error, sometimes chosen on the specious gounds that they are smaller than alternatives such as the standard deviation. This type of presentation is to be avoided since it violates Tufte's principle, in that only two numbers are conveyed with a large amount of ink and any sense of the distribution of the data is lost.

For paired data, scatter plots are useful for verifying the assumptions underlying correlation and regression. In dot plots, where different dots refer to the same individual, as in cross-over trials, it often helps to join the dots.

Graphs are particularly useful in survival data, where a Kaplan-Meier survival plot gives an informative summary of the results.

Analysis

The method of analysis should be clearly described. While t tests and χ^2 tests do not need a reference, anything more complex should have a reference to the relevant methodology. A statistical package that is used should be referenced. It is useful to give the test statistic, degrees of freedom and the exact P value (to no more than two significant figures), since this will enable the reader to judge if the tests have been applied correctly. Thus to compare two proportions one might state ($X^2 = 3.84$, df $= 1$, P $= 0.05$). This tells the reader the type of test (chi-squared), and the exact p value (note that for the result of a chi-squared test the Roman X is used rather than the Greek χ, which refers to the theoretical distribution). Stating either P $=$ NS or P > 0.05 is not recommended, as there is a vast difference in the interpretation of P $= 0.06$ and P $= 0.99$, although they both encompass P > 0.05.

It is a misnomer to refer to "non-parametric data", since it is the statistical test that is non-parametric. Instead one should refer to data that are "not Normally distributed".

1 Gardner M J and Altman D G (eds). *Statistics with confidence.* London: BMJ, 1989.
2 Campbell M J and Machin D. *Medical statistics: a commonsense approach.* 2nd ed. Chichester: John Wiley & Sons, 1993.
3 Tufte E R. *The Visual Display of Quantitative Information.* Cheshire, Connecticut: Graphics Press, 1983.
4 Sleep J and Grant A. West Berkshire perineal management trial: three year follow up. *BMJ,* 1987; **295:** 749–51.

14 Use electronic mail

M S Buckingham

Information may be transmitted from one person to another in a number of ways. Talking face-to-face is informative, direct, and immediate, but may be inconvenient. Talking by telephone is also immediate, but is slightly less informative and may entail delay while the second party is located. Writing is much slower but has the advantage of providing "hard copy", which may be filed and used for future reference. This is important for continuing patient management and for legal purposes. Until recent years good communication between hospital and community depended on a combination of these systems of communication. Hospital information systems and the associated technologies are beginning to add new dimensions to communication.

The modern office

Word processors and personal computers with a wide range of facilities—editing, data storage and retrieval, graphics, formation and duplication of documents—are now very widely used. They do not have to be isolated units. Because these machines can retain the information typed or drawn into them this information can be transmitted to a second word processor or computer via the hospital information system. Outside the hospital, the telephone system may be used. The transmission of information in this way, without paper being physically moved from place to place, is called electronic mail. Electronic mail is immediate, can provide hard copy, and is also flexible, allowing messages to be stored until it is convenient for them to be received.

A number of electronic mail systems have been in use for some years. Telex (short for *tele*printer *ex*change) has been used for many years, but is slow for both sender and recipient, and is not very versatile. Facsimile (fax) transmission is now in general use; it is very quick and diagrams can be transmitted, but the hard copy tends to fade. Computer-to-computer transmission is also very quick, and allows information to be stored and produced as high-quality hard copy when required.

For the purposes of electronic mail within a health district the hardware that constitutes a hospital information system may be used. If such a system is to be established, compatible terminals will need to be sited at all participating centres and offices throughout the district.

Using the system

In the mid-1980s the Winchester Health District introduced the British Telecom Merlin business system on a limited basis into the district general hospital with terminals in a number of general practice surgeries. However, the system was introduced with staff who were far from computer literate; great problems were encountered and over a period of about 18 months the system was abandoned. At about this time a comprehensive main force hospital information system was introduced, using IBM personal computers as terminals. These appeared throughout the hospital, and although there was considerable antipathy initially, the technology is now accepted and is generally thought to be helpful, albeit with some deficiencies remaining. The system continues to evolve. The addition of Windows-based software incorporating word processing and electronic mail is now in widespread use. These enable everybody with access to a terminal and a personal access code to send documents and messages from terminal to terminal.

Within the hospital, the existing information system has permitted messages to be sent from terminal to terminal. The new system will allow this to occur more quickly. In addition, direct communication between the wards and the laboratories and x-ray departments will speed the transmission of information. Communications throughout the district will improve enormously. A number of health centres and surgeries can already receive electronic mail from the hospital information system. For example, discharge summaries can be sent directly from the ward to the surgery and can be printed; deaths and attendances by patients at the accident and emergency department can be notified direct to general practitioners; and daily details of inpatients can be transmitted so that the general practitioner knows which patients are in hospital, how long they have been there, and in which bed they are situated.

In the near future general practitioners will be able to make requests of the laboratories and x-ray departments in the same way as doctors within the hospital. Results of samples sent to the laboratory will be available via the electronic mail system the same day. The efficiency that such a system will provide will be very attractive to purchasers and is appropriately timed to coincide with a combined hospital–community trust.

Beyond communication with the general practitioners will be the links with the family health services authority via the Hampshire County Council electronic mail network. This will allow information pertaining to patient requirements after discharge from hospital to be sent directly to the local department of social services. Support for the patient at home may thus be initiated more efficiently and effectively.

Confidentiality of information is absolutely essential. Access to the mail system is by personal access code number, and information sent from the hospital to non-medical sites is edited appropriately. It is in everybody's interest that sensitive information is treated with the utmost discretion.

Conclusions

Winchester Health District's initial experience with electronic mail was not a conspicuous success. Subsequently, a hospital information system was introduced with less difficulty. It is now so well known and familiar to staff that an extensive electronic mail system has been introduced with a minimum of discomfort.

Acknowledgements

My thanks to Mr Alan Jones, Director of Information Technology, and Dr M du Boulay for technical advice, and to Mrs Pauline Lake for typing the manuscript.

15 Prepare a lecture

R Shields

Most of us receive an invitation to deliver a lecture with some pleasure. After all, it is an opportunity to speak at length, usually without interruption, to an audience of whom at least some wish to hear what we have to say. Unfortunately the audience may not share the pleasure. All too often the invitation is slipped into a drawer and little thought given to the lecture until a few days beforehand. Speakers who assume that a carousel of hastily prepared slides and the mellifluence of their voice will see them through will leave the audience ill-informed and dissatisfied, convinced that the hour devoted to the lecture could have been better spent. It is not trite to say that time spent preparing a lecture is never wasted.

The preparation of a lecture begins with the acceptance of the invitation. You must find out what your host expects and what the members of your audience are looking for—a description of your own research, a general review of recent advances, or a detailed description of practical procedures. What is the mix of the audience? Is there a predominant group with specific objectives—for example, to pass an examination? The most difficult and challenging lecture is without doubt one to a mixed audience, for example an inaugural lecture by a new professor to the staff of a large university, or a presidential lecture to a medical society when spouses and lay guests are present.

Title

Usually you will be asked to give a title when you accept the invitation so that the lecture can be widely advertised. The title should be informative, clearly defining the scope of the lecture. Avoid the vague, whimsical title, which conveys little or nothing to the potential audience. Try in the title to indicate your approach: whether didactic (for example, describing a procedure), provocative (reviewing current concepts and advances), or philosophical (viewing the topic in a much wider context than, for example, merely clinical). The title should be crisp, but not so brief that it does not indicate for whom the lecture is intended. In short, a title should have punch.

Content

In deciding what you are going to say, it is often valuable to define how your lecture would differ from a written communication for a medical journal. A lecture affords you certain opportunities. A lecture can be enhanced by the personality of the speaker, who by his or her enthusiasm can stimulate the audience. Difficult, or contentious, points can be repeated for emphasis, in a way that is not acceptable in a written communication. You can readily express opinions. You may speculate. You can present hypotheses that you would not wish to commit to paper. Results of unpublished or incomplete work can be described. These features can be contained within a lecture and may add to its enjoyment by providing a personal flavour. On the other hand, a written publication quite properly contains long descriptions of methodology and statistical analyses, complex tables, and graphs, all of which would be out of place in a lecture. Too much information should be avoided.

Prune the draft lecture ruthlessly. You are the expert, and your knowledge and experience are greater than that of most of the audience, who can easily be lost or bored with minutiae. Try to limit yourself to one or two aspects of the subject and avoid an encyclopaedic coverage.

You will have to keep within a time limit. For most lectures an hour is set aside, but you should plan to speak for no more than 40-45 minutes.

At this stage you should discuss the scope and content of your lecture with a sympathetic colleague, preferably someone who could be a member of the audience. Try to find out what he or she would look for in the lecture: ask him or her to identify deficiencies in knowledge, so that you will know what to include to give your audience an elementary grasp of the subject.

Form

A lecture must be seen to possess a structure, so that the audience can more readily follow in the direction that you hope to lead them. Various formats are acceptable, but at the very least it should have an introduction, the main body of the lecture, and a conclusion.

Introduction

The introduction has several uses. It enables the members of the audience to get to know you. They can become adjusted to your voice and hopefully to your manner. The introduction also allows you to become acquainted with the size and disposition of the audience in the room. You must try immediately to capture the audience's attention.

You should design your introduction to put forward several important points—the problem areas in the subject should be defined and the objectives that you are setting for yourself outlined. In preparing the introduction you should aim to stimulate the audience, prepare it for the main message, supply the basic information for an understanding of the subject, and establish a relationship with the audience.

There are many ways of introducing the lecture—by an historical allusion, by reference to previous speakers, by an anecdote, even by a provocative statement. You should aim for maximum impact. Occasionally with eponymous lectures, you are expected to allude to the person, or organisation, whom the lecture commemorates. This should always be done, but without obsequiousness or embarrassment to the audience. The link between the lecture and the person it commemorates should not be convoluted. For example, a link between John Hunter and monoclonal antibodies is not immediately apparent to most people: you should avoid too strained an allusion.

A successful introduction will leave the audience wishing, indeed demanding, to hear more.

The main body of the lecture

In preparing the body, or main message, of the lecture, there are several points that you should consider.

Structure

Let the audience perceive the structure of the main part of your lecture. The format can be variable: for example, methods, results, conclusions; or review of published work, your own experience, discussion of your own results and those of others, and general applications. If you clearly demonstrate to the audience that there is order and structure to your lecture, you can take them with you.

Pace

It is in the middle part of a lecture that the skill and experience of a speaker become apparent. The audience, we assume, has been attracted by the title and stimulated by the introduction. There is a risk, however, that about 20 minutes into the lecture its attention will begin to flag. The experienced lecturer, while keeping to the overall plan, should be prepared to vary the pace of the lecture at this point. Avoid proceeding too rapidly into the unfamiliar. You must prepare your lecture to allow yourself some flexibility, so that you can react with the audience—perhaps recapitulating facts previously mentioned, or recalling knowledge already familiar to the audience. Be prepared to break the direction and thrust of the lecture by an anecdote or provocative statement. It is important for the speaker to be aware of this mid-lecture dip in interest. You must not be too rigid or restricted in what you are going to say.

You should consider introducing a change in pace in the second half of the lecture; perhaps be more philosophical, perhaps retain the illustrations for this part of the lecture. You should lead your audience towards the crescendo which forms the conclusion of the lecture.

To read or not to read

You will have to decide whether to speak freely or to read from a script. The introduction and conclusion should be carefully prepared, scripted, and rehearsed; for the main body of the lecture, the structure and salient points only should be memorised. Usually, it is better to speak freely. In this way you can look at the faces in the audience as you speak, and determine whether they are, as you hope, expectant and interested or, unhappily, bored and inattentive. With the printed paper in front of you, you may not respond to the audience. The read lecture can be enthralling, but considerable skill is required in its delivery. Much depends on the importance of the message and the personality of the speaker. The disadvantage of the read lecture is that lecturers may speak monotonously into the lectern, giving the audience the impression that they do not wish to make any contact. Lecturers may be so bound to the printed page that they are afraid to free themselves to move from the lectern to point out salient features of the slides. Sometimes even the speaker begins to sound bored with the lecture.

If you write out the entire text of the lecture to have it before you, you must appreciate the differences between the spoken and written words. In speaking, words are simple and sentences short and of simple construction. If you wish to speak from a written script, read it out several times to others, or into a tape recorder, and modify it until it flows as easily and naturally as the spoken word. Delivery of the written word requires considerable skill and rehearsal to ensure that pauses and changes of pace are included, and natural gestures introduced.

My advice is to speak, rather than read, a lecture. Notes or cards can be prepared as *aides-mémoire*. The text of these should be as concise and brief as possible. You must be familiar with them, so that when you consult them there will not be an embarrassing pause while you try to decipher the writing, or reacquaint yourself with a new theme in your lecture. The typescript should be clear and written only on one side, each card clearly numbered. Thick wads of notes, or a sheaf of galley proofs, can be most offputting to the audience.

Illustrations

Speakers who graduate from the 10–15 minute paper to the 50-minute lecture may conclude that if 10 slides are appropriate for a short communication, 40–50 slides are necessary for a lecture. Slides, projected every minute in a darkened or semidarkened room will leave even the most interested audience asleep within 15 minutes. Good slides, the design and content of which are a task in themselves, should preferably be projected in sequences, so that the lights are not being continually switched on and off in a distracting manner during the lecture. Slides, videotapes, and films may be kept to the latter half of the lecture, when the audience's interest may be flagging. Slides should not be used to jog the memory of the lecturer, but to emphasise the spoken word, to provide the audience with a visual memory, or perhaps, to show them in an illustration something that would take some time to describe in words. Unfortunately, slides are often used by nervous and insecure lecturers as a blanket to insulate themselves from the audience.

There is, today, an increasing vogue for double projection. In expert hands, with, say, one slide displaying a concept and the other details, this technique can produce excellent results. Frequently, it is just a device to swamp the audience with even more detail. Lecturers should not attempt double projection in a lecture room, or with equipment, with which they are not familiar.

Conclusion

You must clearly define the conclusion of your lecture, not just stop talking. The conclusion should be well prepared, rehearsed, and come over in a crisp, upbeat manner. Remember that the audience often feels pleased and satisfied if you return to concepts and ideas mentioned in the introduction. An audience likes to feel that, at least for the moment, the subject has been wrapped up. Do not include new facts or concepts in your conclusion. However you choose to conclude, the audience should be made aware that you are concluding: you should finish strongly, almost inviting the audience to break out into spontaneous applause.

Immediate preparations

You can very often allay the nervousness that you may feel, and increase your confidence that nothing will go wrong, by careful preparation immediately before giving the lecture. You must ask your host to let you see the lecture room beforehand. Look at the disposition of seats, whether you have to extend your neck to deliver your words to the back of highly tiered seats or to throw them to the back of a flat room. Check the acoustics. Try if possible not to use the microphone but if you must, use one that is held around the neck rather than fixed, so that you can walk from the lectern to the screen. What is the lectern like? Some are simple; others with buttons, switches, and dials resemble the flight deck of Concorde. Become familiar with the essential switches. Make sure that you are not obscured by a large lectern—and be prepared to step aside from it, particularly during the introduction and conclusion. Look at the relative positions of the lectern and screen, for you must avoid running back and forward between them during the course of the lecture. Have a test slide projected to check that you can see it easily and not have to crane your neck to do so. Decide who will change the slides—yourself or a projectionist—and give the projectionist clear instructions about switching lights on and off. It is usually useful to have, as the first slide in the carousel, one that can be used exclusively for focusing and is unrelated to the rest of the lecture, so that you do not have to show the audience your first slide, which is usually one with some impact.

Look for pitfalls—a narrow platform, stairs, wires, stools that you may fall over or down. Check how to operate overhead projectors and videotape films. If you are going to use the blackboard, see that chalk and duster are available. Check that there is a pointer and, if it is an electric one, determine how it works and particularly out of which end the light comes. Remind yourself to put the pointer down when not in use. There is nothing more distracting to an audience than to have the red spot of a laser beam dancing over the ceiling and the members of the audience.

Preparing oneself

Of all the preparations, perhaps the most difficult, is of yourself. Remember that a feeling of tension and nervousness is a frequent accompaniment of any major performance. Once you get into the body of the lecture and talking about a subject that interests you, your nervousness will go. Many accomplished lecturers would be concerned if they did not experience some tension beforehand.

We have enjoyed memorable lectures delivered by highly skilled and polished speakers. There are those who possess acting skills, and who, by gestures, pauses, and force of delivery, can capture and retain the attention of the audience. These skills are usually acquired by experience—by careful preparation and rehearsal, and by clear-sighted analysis of each lecture after it has been given, to determine how it might be modified in the future.

A lecture is a bit of a performance, quite a challenging one because you have to write the script as well as deliver the lines. Remember that the members of the audience have usually come of their own accord and, at least initially, will be on your side. If you are speaking on a subject on which you have knowledge, and radiate your enthusiasm, if you show that you have given your lecture careful preparation and quickly establish a rapport with your audience, you will be successful in making the audience enjoy itself and receptive to the new concepts and information. The time spent in preparation will have made the lecture worthwhile both to you and to the audience.

16 Give a lecture

Richard Leech

> Speak the speech, I pray you . . .
> William Shakespeare, *Hamlet*

Contrary to popular belief, the gifts of the actor, such as they are, are quite different to the gift of the gab. The trouble is that, although I have picked up a few wrinkles on making myself heard in public over the past 40 years, I have previously had the benefit of cleverer and more articulate fellows to write the words. It's a different kettle of fish when you have to make it up yourself.

However, needs must when the devil and the *BMJ* drive. I have lately done a bit of research and studied the form at a few centres of postgraduate learning. This is quite simple nowadays, for since the minister has seen fit to award a bonus to general practitioners who attend such centres there has been a mushroom growth. There is hardly a hospital in the kingdom now that doesn't shove out the postgraduate boat—often loaded to the scuppers with goodies from the drug companies.

I have been amazed to discover how few of the lecturers at these establishments have bothered to consider the basic principles of voice production and presentation: principles without which no actor would ever achieve his or her first job. Thus I have been encouraged to believe that I have something to tell you that may be of help. I am not concerned with what you say. You have had expert advice on how to marshal your facts. I am only presuming to offer a few hints on how to say them.

First of all, then, you need to take up a position in good light where you can be comfortably seen by every member of the audience. Actors know all about this. It is a truism to say that selfish actors grab the centre of the stage. But they do it for the very good reason that it is the easiest place from which to command an audience. As far as possible they will speak "out front" rather than "up stage" or "into the wings". If they can, they will avoid speaking on the move. These are not arbitrary fashions. They are immutable laws which actors break at their peril.

In my researches I have discovered that many lecturers bury their heads in their notes, quickly narcotising their audience by having an intimate love affair with their own handwriting. With confidence born of thorough rehearsal, it should not be necessary to consult notes, unless the performer is using them as a device to enable him to draw aside and let a particular passage sink home. You remember Antony in his funeral oration:

"My heart is in the coffin there with Caesar,
And I must pause till it come back to me."

The actor who carries the book on stage is unlikely to win any awards, but for doctors, who after all have other more pressing calls on their time than the perfection of the actor's art, notes may be excused. But they must be used as memory aids and not read from. One topic ended, lecturers should drop their head, read in silence, compose their new thoughts, then lift their head and continue.

There is a particular danger in case history notes. I came upon many doctors who were doing very nicely until they came to illustrating their point by reference to case notes. These notes record a particular triumph of diagnosis or treatment; otherwise the doctors wouldn't have bothered to bring them. But they have forgotten the details. That's why they need the notes. As they refresh their memory, they become fascinated by their own past brilliance, totally forget the audience, and, with nose deep in the notes, lapse into mumbling anecdotage.

Talking up stage

I am deaf and depend heavily on lip-reading, so I am particularly harassed by a performer who turns away. But even for people with the ears of an elk hound, lip-reading plays a part, as does facial expression, and communication is restricted when the head is turned away. There are occasions when it is unavoidable—for example, drawing on a blackboard or demonstrating the details on a slide. Actors call it "talking up stage", and when they can't escape it they make a particular effort to lift their voice and project more clearly in order to overcome it.

The pointer is another hazard that encourages the exhibition of the Dick Whittington syndrome. This is where lecturers shoulder the pointer and set out on the last ten miles for London, becoming so engrossed in the route march that they lose the audience by the way.

Many postgraduate centres are now equipped with microphones, but unless you are lecturing in a football field it is possible to do without them. Indeed, for all but experts they are apt to do more harm than good. The major danger, I think, is the temptation to use the microphone as a charm that will ward off evil and magically transform an unconfident, ill-prepared mumbling attack of verbal diarrhoea into an interesting and audible discourse. I have seen—I can't say heard—many performers groaning away, making not even the natural effort they would to speak across a room, in the complacent belief that the microphone is transforming all. If you use a microphone, you have to speak into it from a distance that remains nearly constant. Rapid variation in the distance causes electronic thunderstorms. This problem can be overcome by a chest mike —which should be hung six to nine inches from the mouth. I sat under a London consultant lately who inherited the chest mike from a Scottish giant, and failed to adjust the neck strap. The instrument hung like a string of bones round a witch doctor's neck. It may have worked like a charm for him, but it didn't help us, and after a while we even gave up listening to the borborygmi. The chest mike can add a complication to the Dick Whittington syndrome if you allow the lead to get tangled up with your legs.

Breath the creator

In the beginning was the word. But in order to transmit it you need breath. Breath is the great creator. God breathed on a handful of dust to create man. It is impossible to exaggerate the importance of filling the lungs with air. A chestful of air is a wonderful antidote to butterflies in the stomach. That ghastly moment when you stand surveying the many-headed monster, courage oozing from the heels of your shoes, can be converted to a moment of confidence if you stop worrying and concentrate on taking a really deep breath.

Good breathing automatically neutralises a whole catalogue of faults—for example, the infuriating lack of communication that results from dropping the ends of sentences. This is caused by a dwindling in the supply of air in the lungs, until there is no longer enough to carry the sound away and so it drowns in a gurgle in the throat. Actors use this shortage of breath to effect. We call it "throwing away a line", and lots of consultants I heard are on to it. It can be a witty, sophisticated effect. But, as Nöel Coward said, if you're throwing a line away, you need to be quite sure where you are throwing it. Though it should come across as an aside—an afterthought or snide comment on your own lecture—it is, of course, totally valueless unless it is heard.

In a brief tip-sheet of the most obvious faults of voice production, I have only space for one more. It is the question of where you "place" your voice, how you use—or fail to use—the resonant cavities of your head. Some lucky people place their voices naturally forward in the front of the mouth and their words wing happily to their audience. But others keep the sound trapped in the back of their throat, a fault exaggerated by the tightened muscles of nervousness. It is a particularly English complaint. Celts tend not to be so afflicted. In extreme cases you get the state of affairs celebrated in the story about the New York barman who said to his visitor, "Say, you're English, aren't ya?" and the stranger replied, "If I were any more English I couldn't talk at all."

It is a fault more difficult to eradicate than most others. Sufferers tend not to be able to distinguish the difference in placing. Once you can hear the difference, you can't bear to make the mistake. Chronic sufferers really need expert advice, but a brief first-aid treatment, that has helped me, is to repeat, "Teeth—lips—tip of the tongue" over and over, at the same time trying to feel the resonance in your antra and the front of your face.

17 Lecture abroad

David Lowe

Unless you think, like Nancy Mitford, that "abroad is unutterably bloody", you will want to be asked to lecture overseas. You will be flattered at the invitation, excited by the prospect of travel to foreign parts, game enough to suffer at least a little discomfort, and faintly nervous at what you might be letting yourself in for.

Abroad is not homogeneous: the problems you may face in the United States will be different from the problems of going to parts of Asia. Some of the potential difficulties are discussed below.

Paperwork

The first hurdle is usually to get permission to go. If you are employed by the NHS, there will be forms to apply for study leave approval, and you may need to arrange cover with colleagues or locums. University employees may need the consent of their dean and head of department as well.

Permission to visit may be needed from the host country. Visas should be applied for early: some consulates take weeks to process applications. If you are visiting a country such as Pakistan or Egypt at the invitation of the armed forces, they are often able to expedite matters and will be disappointed not to be asked. On the visa application form you should state that you will be giving lectures, teaching, or taking part in a conference (in addition to any sightseeing), as this may determine the type of visa that you are given. You might not be allowed to accept a fee for a lecture if a work visa has not been issued.

Most travel insurance policies do not make separate provision for travel abroad for work rather than tourism but it is worth checking this. It is essential to have medical insurance even if you are the guest of the ministry of health in the host country. If you are ill, the local facilities may be able to cope, but *in extremis* you may have to be flown home. Advice on prophylaxis against malaria and immunisation against other infectious diseases abroad can be obtained by telephone from British Airways travel centres. Many general practitioners subscribe to a software update that is also very informative on the current state of malaria, yellow fever, cholera, and other infectious diseases.

Planning and packing

If you are invited somewhere you have not visited, try to speak to someone who has been there. Your hosts or your royal college may be able to give you names of previous lecturers. If you can find out what the accommodation and transport arrangements in the host country are likely to be, you will be able to plan your packing better. A small water-heater and a shortwave radio can make even the most desperate facilities bearable.

Try to agree what the procedural arrangements will be before you go. Planning obviously relies on efficient communications. I once received a letter regretting that my trip had been cancelled four days after my planned departure date. Find out the address and telephone number of the place in which you will be staying so that you can be contacted if an emergency arises at home.

Let your hosts know the date and time of your arrival and the airline you will be using. You may wish to be independent and make your own way from the airport to the venue, but in some countries this is unwise and in a few it may be dangerous, especially after dark. Try to arrange for someone to meet you.

You can find out what type of climate and temperatures to expect from the broadsheet newspapers. The intensity of your hotel heating or air conditioning may come as a shock: you can swelter in a Scandinavian winter and shiver in a subtropical summer. The first is easily accommodated by shedding layers of clothing, but you should consider packing a light jumper or cardigan if you go somewhere hot.

Arranging the lectures

Some hosts arrange broad timings for lecture courses but, out of courtesy, leave the details to the lecturer. If you are unaware of this, you might find that the day of your arrival is spent drawing up a programme. Where possible, the course contents and sequence of lectures should be agreed with your hosts and any other visiting lecturers before you go. For example, say that you understand you will be staying in a certain hotel or hostel, lecturing for so many hours, having this or that day free, and returning on a particular date. Even so, your programme is likely to become distorted because start times are delayed, lunches are extended, and transport does not arrive.

How you lecture will depend on the audience that you will be addressing. If it is not obvious, ask your hosts whether the audience will consist of medical students or postgraduates, generalists or specialists, and whether spouses, non-medical staff, or the press will be invited. (In some countries members of the press are invited to national and international meetings as a matter of course and not, deflatingly, because they have been alerted that you will be appearing.) You may need to be careful of the images that you project and possibly the language that you use if non-medical people will be present.

Terminology differs among countries. You can look up terms in a textbook in the host country's language. For example, the French and Russians are fond of eponyms, and the names might not be the ones that you are used to. In Britain we refer to the Circle of Willis, but the French, with more geometrical nicety, call it the Polygon.

Audiovisual material

The visual and other material that you take will be determined by your style of lecturing, the information that you wish to convey, and the facilities available at your venue. The equipment can vary from a blackboard without chalk to a three-projector split screen *son et lumière* with independent/simultaneous advance and reverse (if you are given the choice, find the chalk!). Facilities for slides and overhead projection will usually be available, but the slide-carrier may not be the one you expect. In a humid climate, glass mounted slides can develop condensation which might boil from the heat of a powerful projector lamp and spoil the acetate.

Lecture notes or handouts prepared before you go will almost always be of better quality than ones photocopied immediately before a lecture, and they do not usually weigh much. When large numbers are needed, your hosts may prefer to help with postage or excess baggage charges on the flight rather than undertake to reproduce a top copy on your arrival.

Foreign currency

If at all possible you must buy foreign currency before you go. No matter how well organised a trip is, you may find that you have to take a taxi or pay for a meal or drinks because of an unscheduled delay. Some currencies are difficult to obtain so apply to your bank or travel agent as soon as your departure date is confirmed. If you are going to a country with non-negotiable currency, take dollar notes. If you plan to use a credit or charge card to pay for accommodation or other expenses abroad, check that it will be accepted; even large hotels will sometimes not honour certain cards.

Hospitality abroad is often generous. You might consider taking some small gifts for your hosts, their secretaries, or the car driver. Simple, small, and specific items go down well, such as a mug or T-shirt with the logo of your medical college or professional association. Only give a royal college or other attributable tie if you are sure that the recipient is permitted to wear it; your innocent presentation may be misconstrued as official and committing.

Travelling out

In concrete rather than allegorical terms, the saying "to travel hopefully is a better thing than to arrive" is rubbish. It is much better to arrive, and preferably on time. On the day you set off on your trip remember the three most important reasons for frustration and disappointment: delay, delay, and delay. You could use the time to catch up on your reading, assess papers, write book reviews, or draft grant applications. This should confound your detractors who think that lecturing overseas is a holiday. Take your slides and other lecture material as hand luggage if possible. Then, if your suitcase is delivered to the wrong side of the world, you can still give your lecture.

Jet lag can be incapacitating after long journeys. If it is likely to be a problem, try to arrange at least one free day at the start of your engagements to recover. Human beings have a "natural" day of 25

101

hours; jet lag is therefore said to be less when you travel west. I have never found that this made much difference.

Lecturing

There are some points worth considering when you are delivering a lecture to an audience whose language and idiom are not your own:

(1) Speak slowly. This is more difficult than you might think, especially as you will be enthusiastic about your subject. Watch your audience's faces—they will tell you when you are wasting their time and yours.

(2) Leave your slides up longer. If the participants are reading and copying from them, they may need more time than you think. Consider reproducing the written material on the slides as handouts, so that the audience can concentrate on what you are saying.

(3) Keep the content of the slides to a minimum. If necessary, use more slides. Identify the areas that you are talking about with a pointer.

(4) Say what you are going to say, say it, and then say what you have said.

(5) Avoid idiomatic phrases, complex sentences, and unusual words. Don't take this to extremes. If you analyse each sentence before you deliver it, you'll sound awkward and unnatural.

(6) Don't lecture in a foreign language unless you are fluent. It is upsetting to have the audience giggling at your gaucheries.

(7) Don't tell jokes or use irony unless you are absolutely sure of your audience. At best they may not understand and at worst they will take you seriously.

(8) Avoid politics. Depending on where you are, this can be embarrassing and sometimes dangerous.

These points are still relevant if you speak British English and your audience speaks American, Canadian, or Indian English, for example, and vice versa: perhaps more so, as you may have an unrealistic sense of well-being.

Some concepts do not translate well. An English friend of mine, speaking in his clipped received pronunciation in the United States, started his lectures with a slide that read "Yes, I really do speak like this all the time" and got a laugh. He tried it in South America to a predominantly English-speaking audience, and was surprised to get a bigger laugh from the Brazilians: it was translated into "in reality I say this sort of thing interminably."

In many parts of the world medicine is taught in English, but in continental Europe, the Far East, and South America you will be given an interpreter. This is a very mixed blessing. Sequential interpretation disjoints a lecture. Simultaneous interpretation allows you to lecture relatively normally, but the faster you speak the more rudimentary the interpretation will be, and there may be mistakes. There may also be a small, tinny voice audible from a nearby set of headphones that stops a second or two after you, which can be very distracting. Give the interpreter a copy of your lecture the day before. You will not, of course, deliver it word for word, but it will give him or her an idea of the contents and of the vocabulary that you are likely to use.

Slides made in the language and script of the host country can be used as a courtesy to start or summarise a lecture. Most hospitals have a list of people who will act as translators; consulates can often supply names of professionals whose charges are reasonable. Modern word-processing software will supply Cyrillic, Greek, and Hebrew characters.

When you leave your hotel each day take with you more material than you think you will need, and be prepared to use less than you had planned. There will be occasions when a lecturer who should speak before you cannot attend, and others when the audience wishes to explore a particular point for longer than you had expected. You may also find that you are collected from your hotel with fellow lecturers and have to wait for some time before your turn, so take a book.

Coming home

Payment for the work and reimbursement of expenses are usually arranged at the end of the visit. The formalities can take hours. If you are to be paid soft or local currency rather than sterling or dollars, check that you will be able to convert it at the airport or through your bank at home. You may be better buying goods and exporting them instead.

Travelling home may be more frustrating than travelling out. Delays seem worse because you are looking forward to seeing your family and friends again. The duty-free shop may be a disappointment, and you will have spent or changed back all of your local currency and have no hope of buying a cup of tea from the airport café. But you will almost certainly have enjoyed yourself, and when the invitation comes to lecture abroad again next year you will leap at it.

- Speak slowly
- Show slides slowly
- Limit the content of slides
- Stand up, speak up, shut up
- Don't use idioms and unusual words
- Leave time for questions
- Don't lecture in a foreign language if you don't have to
- Be careful with jokes
- Avoid politics

18 Devise a course for overseas visitors who don't speak English well

B B Seedhom, J E Smeathers, D T Thompson

Running a residential course requires thorough planning. This is particularly so when the delegates are from a country where the first language is not English. A group from the rheumatism research unit in Leeds recently ran such a course. The subject was biomechanics, particularly of the knee, and the audience was a group of orthopaedic surgeons from Japan who visited this country for 12 days. The need for such a course had been firmly identified, and it was seen as an opportunity to form links between us and the medical profession in Japan while raising funds for the unit. This chapter describes the problems we found, the strategies we adopted, and our successes (and failures) in presenting this particular course.

Aims of the course

Persuading a group of professionals to devote considerable time and money to a course requires that a definite need for the course has been established. In our case this was identified on a paper describing the state of biomechanical research in orthopaedics in Japan.[1] The paper was based on a questionnaire sent to medical schools in Japan with orthopaedic departments. One of the conclusions was that "the majority of (Japanese) orthopaedists involved in bioengineering research feel the lack of engineering knowledge and technique and have a desire to gain such knowledge". We decided that a short, intensive bioengineering course on a subject of mutual interest would be attractive to Japanese surgeons.

The aims of the course must be made clear, and all organisers must be aware of them. It is best to start with organisational aims—namely, why and how you intend to run the course—and work down to the specific educational aims. These should be written down and circulated for discussion. Some members of the team may well disagree with the aims. If their objections cannot be overcome by discussion, they may decide not to contribute. This can be disappointing, but it is far better to find out at this stage than to produce, after days of preparation, material that is inconsistent.

The aims of the bioengineering course were split into two groups. The organisational aims were: to form links with the orthopaedic profession in Japan; to raise funds for the research unit; and to provide an attractive package comprising both technical education and recreation. The educational aims were: to ensure that the participants left with some working knowledge of the fundamentals of engineering mechanics and materials science on which orthopaedic biomechanics is based; to provide an insight into the way engineers in general, and bioengineers in particular, approach a problem; to provide a series of lectures on a particular topic of bioengineering to illustrate this; and to make the surgeons aware of the work in progress in the major centres of bioengineering in Great Britain.

Anticipated problems and preparation

When delegates commit themselves to the expense of time away from work, and possibly a long overseas journey, the organisers are under a heavy obligation to provide a professional service. Most of this is to do with attention to detail: clearly presented lectures, well maintained and tested equipment, comfortable lecture theatres, adequate meals and accommodation, and efficient transport. None of these is appreciably different from the problems encountered in organising any residential course. It is important, however, to try to predict problems specific to the particular course and audience, especially any problems related to language.

All the surgeons on our course could read and write English. Most, however, were not used to assimilating spoken English. Our previous experience with Japanese visitors to the unit had made us aware that the normal type of lecture presentation would not be adequate. The problems of communicating with an audience in a language other than their own were exacerbated in this case by the need for specialist terminology. Much of this—for example, the terms "stress" and "strain"—causes particular problems owing to the confusion of meaning between uses in the engineering and medical professions.

As far as the engineering course was concerned, it was not easy to predict how familiar the participants would be with the concepts of engineering mechanics. It was, therefore, difficult to decide at what level it would be appropriate to start this part of the course. It is our experience that mechanical concepts are really appreciated only when they are applied in solving problems. Without a grasp of these concepts, the students would be unable to appreciate fully the specialist lectures in the course. We were concerned, however, about the reaction of a group of surgeons to an "examples class" approach, where they would be asked to make calculations and answer questions reinforcing the main points of the previous lecture.

Many of the group would be visiting Britain for the first time. Although they were anxious to make the most of their visit academically, it was clear that filling their available time with lectures alone would be counterproductive. Ideally, they should be able to recover after their journey, be given time to accustom themselves to the language before facing serious academic tasks, and know that there would be adequate time for sightseeing and shopping.

Discussions about the aims and design of the package deal took place roughly one year before the event. From the start one of the organisers was a surgeon in Japan, who looked at our ideas, discussed them with colleagues, and made suggestions. In doing this he also acted as our local advertising agent by bringing the course to the attention of possible delegates.

In consultation with our Japanese colleagues we decided that the right mixture of recreation and education would be achieved with a 14-day package deal. Air travel to and from Tokyo would occupy one day each way, which would allow 12 days in Britain. Most of the academic material would be presented as a three-day intensive course. We decided that the best way of providing an appreciation of current bioengineering research was for the surgeons to visit various well-known centres. The time before and after the course would, therefore, include visits to such centres, as well as providing time for recovery, acclimatisation to the new language, sightseeing, and shopping.

As the package began to take shape it became clear that we needed someone to take responsibility for the travel and accommodation.

TABLE—*Itinerary of fortnight's course on biomechanical engineering for Japanese orthopaedic surgeons*

Day	Day of week	Time	Activity
1	Thursday		Air travel from Tokyo
2	Friday	0605	Arrive Heathrow from Hong Kong; breakfast at Strand Palace Hotel
		1100	Imperial College Bioengineering Centre
3	Saturday		At leisure in London; overnight stay at Strand Palace Hotel
4	Sunday		Journey to Leeds via Cambridge; accommodation at university conference centre
5	Monday		Sightseeing in Yorkshire, Harrogate, Fountains Abbey, and Ripon
6	Tuesday ⎫		
7	Wednesday ⎬		Three-day course
8	Thursday ⎭		
		1700	Conference dinner at Ripon
9	Friday		Journey to Edinburgh via Alnwick, Bamburgh castle, and Lindisfarne
10	Saturday		At leisure in Edinburgh
11	Sunday		Journey to Chester via Moffat and Windermere
12	Monday		Journey to Oxford via Stratford on Avon
13	Tuesday	0900	Nuffield Orthopaedic Engineering Centre, Oxford
		1530	Depart for London; overnight stay at Excelsior Hotel, Heathrow
14	Wednesday	0915	Air travel to Tokyo

Consequently, we appointed a secretary for the equivalent of one day a week for the four months before the event. She was taken on full time during the two-week visit. As the Japanese party signed up for the trip they arranged for a tour guide who could speak English to liaise with us. This guide eventually travelled to Britain with the party and proved invaluable. With hindsight we would strongly recommend this arrangement of secretary and tour guide taking joint responsibility for the organisation of the trip, while a member of the visiting party should be available to advise on the academic aspects of the course.

The size of the party was finalised a month before the event. The detailed itinerary had to be decided on at this stage so that hotel bookings could be made taking advantage of discounts for large parties and early bookings (see table). Hotels were booked close to the bioengineering centres and sightseeing areas that the party wished to visit. The university conference centre at Leeds was booked for the short period of the course. No special meals were requested by the delegates, so traditional English fare was provided throughout their stay. Our visitors did, however, make regular use of local Chinese restaurants.

A luxury coach, which was available for the entire period of the package, was used for transport. Although there were periods when the coach was idle, it had many advantages over alternatives such as trains, hired cars, and local buses. It provided an economical and flexible door-to-door service and so allowed the maximum use of available time with little risk of losing people in transit. The tour guide was able to ensure that overall schedules were maintained while the visitors themselves had considerable control over what they did and saw within that schedule.

Course details

During the planning of the three-day course of lectures it became apparent that the greatest problem of communication was that the students were unfamiliar with spoken English. To assess the magnitude of this problem we performed a full dress rehearsal of the course before the delegates arrived. All the lecturers and demonstrators on the course were present while each lecturer presented his lecture in full. Fortunately, two of the lecturers—an engineer researching into a related subject and an orthopaedic surgeon, both working in the university—were Japanese and thus able to offer helpful comments. Each lecture was evaluated on the basis of content, level of understanding required, structure, clarity of presentation, how the various aids were to be used (slides, models and visual aids), and, most importantly, the language. All idiomatic phrases (well; I am afraid; it is all very well but, etc) had to be omitted. Complex phrases were made much simpler, and a consistent and limited vocabulary was adhered to. Jargon and technical terms were explained as they occurred, and emphasis was placed on diction. It is not easy for a foreigner to understand garbled pronunciation, especially when two or more words have the same sound but completely different meanings. The speed of delivery was also slowed down to that which our Japanese lecturers could follow. We found it helpful if one of the organisers sat at the back of the lecture room as a monitor. His function was to alert the speaker if he spoke too fast or too quietly. The dress rehearsal also enabled us to check the seating arrangements in the lecture theatre and the audiovisual equipment. We considered that uniformity of the seating arrangements was essential. Although this would appear to be an obvious aspect of organising any course, it is seldom paid enough attention. Often there are first and second-class seats: an overhead projector may obscure vision, or its noisy cooling fan may reduce audibility. To avoid these problems each seat was examined individually for clarity of sight and sound. Projectors were placed as far back as possible to reduce the noise (this, of course, would not be a problem in a purpose-built auditorium with a separate projection room).

In addition to the slow delivery we decided that a visual display of the key words of each lecture was required. To avoid loss of continuity of the theme of the lecture two slide projectors and screens were used. One screen carried the theme slides while the other carried the key words relevant to the slide. A booklet was provided that included the same list of key words so that the delegate could find the correct page at any time by comparing the listed key words with those on the screen. The booklet contained space for the student to take notes about each concept. Other audiovisual materials were used only when absolutely necessary—for instance, overhead projectors were used for graphs, and previously prepared diagrams and working models were used to provide tangible evidence of the concepts being discussed. Video tapes were used to show points of interest and concepts that could not be readily shown in the lecture room.

The core of the course was a series of specialist lectures about biomechanical aspects of the human knee joint, its kinematic function, loading and force transmission, commonly occurring damage, and techniques of surgical repair and prosthetic replacement of the knee. To appreciate this material fully a working knowledge of the concepts of bioengineering was required. We also needed to ensure that the audience had a common level of understanding of these concepts. The specialist lectures on the knee were, therefore, interwoven with a series of "service lectures" that provided this theoretical background. The theory was made relevant by closely tailoring each service lecture to the needs of the following specialist lecture. Similarly, the topics of the specialist lectures were presented in such a sequence that the teaching of engineering concepts could be developed in a structured way. At crucial points in the development of the theory the lectures were supplemented with examples classes. These were designed both to give the delegates the opportunity to exercise the analytical tools that they were being introduced to and to allow us to monitor the progress of the students

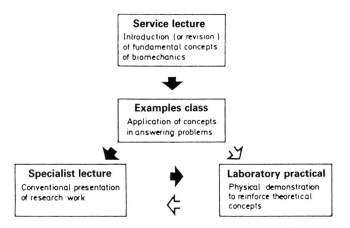

Generalised strategy of lecture presentation showing how each specialist lecture was supported by extra lectures and preparation work.

to ensure that the lectures were being presented at the appropriate level. The figure shows the hierarchy of the various types of lectures used during the course.

Appraisal of the course

It is instructive and valuable to know for future reference how successful the course was through discussion with all those who participated. A good structure for this is to work through original aims and assess how successful the course was in achieving each goal. It is also useful if all participants make a written list of what they consider were the successes and failures. A questionnaire given to the delegates before they leave may be helpful. If this is to be of value, it must be well thought out and the time required to prepare it not underestimated.[2] It must be prepared in advance of the course and be ready for the audience immediately the course ends.

An interactive approach has several advantages. We drew several conclusions about our course from discussions with the delegates. The course was very favourably received. Many delegates admitted that they had had low expectations of how much they would be able to learn because of the communication problem but that they had been pleasantly surprised. The rehearsal of all the service lectures and most of the specialist lectures ensured the smooth running and continuity of the lecture course, the benefits of which were so

111

apparent that we would recommend that this should form an important part of any lecture course. The use of key words on the second projector screen was certainly worth the extra effort required in the presentation. The examples classes were surprisingly successful in that the delegates enjoyed them and often completed them before the end of the session. This may have been helped by the intensely competitive temperament within this particular group. Others benefited from the one-to-one discussion that was possible because of the number of staff available during examples classes.

The prepared notebook was not as well used as had been hoped. It is easy to underestimate the skill required in taking lecture notes, especially when this problem is compounded by the use of a second language. The notebooks did, however, serve as a useful *aide-mémoire* for the delegates to take home with them at the end of the course. Many of the delegates used cameras in the lecture theatre, and some even had miniature tape recorders. Perhaps this easily available technology could be used to reduce the need for taking notes on future courses.

The excursions to places of historical interest were much enjoyed, and the ratio of one academic to two recreational days proved to be an acceptable balance. The tour guide was useful, as he was able to advise us about the major subjects of interest within the touring party, and this resulted in an impromptu trip to St Andrew's golf course. In retrospect, we could have tailored the recreation more closely to the interests of our party if we had contacted the tour guide before their arrival. We certainly underestimated the Japanese interest in golf.

1 Terayama K. The present state of biomechanical research in orthopaedics in Japan—an observation by an orthopaedic surgeon. *Eng Med* 1983; **12**: 207–9.
2 Youngman M B. *Designing and analysing questionnaires*. Nottingham: University of Nottingham, 1978. (Rediguide 12)

19 Use an overhead projector

T S Murray

An overhead projector is now a standard piece of equipment in most teaching departments. This versatile visual aid can be used efficiently if a number of basic rules are followed.

During a lecture the overhead projector may be used to supplement or replace the blackboard. It is clean, provides teachers with an almost limitless area, and allows them to face their audience. The room does not need to be darkened and the flow of presentation is therefore uninterrupted. Lecturers are responsible for their own transparencies and can control the order and timing of presentation of the material. They can also even add to or alter the material during the presentation.

The screen should be mounted as high as possible so that the audience has a clear view. The projector can be placed in the centre with the screen directly facing the audience, or the screen can be placed obliquely in a corner, with the projector in a corresponding position. On a vertical screen a tilted beam of light produces an image that is wider at the top than the bottom (keystone distortion). This effect is prevented by tilting the upper edge of the screen forwards.

Acetate roll

An acetate roll used on the projector provides a large surface area, equivalent to about 50 feet of blackboard. The best results on an acetate roll are obtained by using a technical pen with special ink, which can be either water soluble or permanent. When the page of acetate has been filled, the roll is wound on to reveal a clean surface. Later, the roll can be wound back and used to recap the session if required.

Preparation of transparencies

Transparencies may be used to introduce, illustrate, or consolidate a lecture, and to reinforce the important headings. They can be prepared at short notice (when the production of slides would be impossible), a great advantage when preparation time is limited. Many doctors do not have access to audiovisual departments for producing slides, but can prepare transparencies themselves with minimal materials and reach an acceptable standard if they take care in preparation.

If the transparencies are to form part of a permanent teaching package, it is best to buy a box of acetate sheets. Cellofilm, which is cheaper, can also be used, but it is flimsy and tends to curl when exposed to heat and moisture; x-ray film that has been developed can also be used, the simplest method of cleaning being to soak the sheets in soap and water overnight. If none of these materials is available, polyethylene may be used.

On acetate sheets it is necessary to use special pens, which can have either a spirit base or a water base. The use of water-based pens allows the acetate sheets to be washed and used again, an undoubted advantage when the material is needed on only one occasion—for example, a case presentation. The pens, which are of various thicknesses, can be obtained at a graphics shop, are easy to use, and produce professional-looking transparencies; stencils to use with them are also available. Ordinary pens are unsuitable on acetate but can be used on cellofilm.

Normal typewriter type is too small to produce a satisfactory visual image for transparencies. Even if the height of a letter is increased, type that is 10-12 characters to the inch will appear too crowded. The solution centres on increasing the size of the projected image, and typewriters modified to provide a large character, at a frequency of about six to the inch, are available. Golf-ball typewriters with special heads and personal computers can also produce large characters.

The transparencies are mounted in cardboard to aid storage and prevent damage. The mounts must not interfere with the visual content, and at least 15mm should be left between the inside of the frame and the outer limit of the content. Mounts also aid handling during presentation, and the registration pegs on the projector allow accurate positioning.

The most important aspect of any visual aid is communication with the audience, so the material must be easily understood and legible. If you are unhappy about printing, you can use self-adhesive transfer letters. The whole of the transparency must be in focus; a blurred picture can be the result of dust on the lens and mirror, but a poor transparency is a more likely cause. Information must be restricted to eight words a line and eight lines to a transparency. Use of several different colours can add impact, help to emphasise points, and give variety, and self-adhesive colour films can be used for this purpose.

Anatomical drawings can be traced directly on to acetate by using an episcope, which can reduce or enlarge the size of the drawing by projecting the image. If this equipment is not available, the drawing may be enlarged using the overhead projector itself. Trace the drawing on cellofilm, then project and trace it directly on to acetate. Commercial kits with explicit instructions, such as Letravision, are available and allow a professional transparency to be produced easily and quickly.

Specific techniques

Masking is used for covering information at various stages in a lecture. By using a sheet of plain white paper, lecturers can mask the whole transparency and reclaim the full attention of the class. By moving the paper, they reveal the teaching points one by one. They can read the text through the paper, and thus are in complete control of the presentation and can lead the discussion to a particular point before projecting the next line of notes. Use of the switch can also attract the audience's attention: switch off when you want the attention, and switch on when the attention has to be given to the overhead projection.

A pen may be used to point to a specific part, word, or sentence on a transparency that the lecturer wants to emphasise. The pen must not be waved about, however, as this can be distracting. The pen can also be used to underline points.

Silhouetting can be produced by laying objects on the projector. This often leads to better understanding—for example, of the position of a prosthetic valve during a lecture on cardiac surgery.

Perspex models may also be used in this way to illustrate difficult teaching points—for example, the actions of the intrinsic muscles of the larynx.

Overlays are separate sheets that are placed on top of the main drawing or diagram. They add information and can be used to build up complex diagrams; an overlay showing the system of blood vessels, for example, can be placed over a diagram of a limb, and this could be followed by an overlay showing the peripheral nerve supply. Several different commercially prepared transparencies and overlays are available in all medical subjects.

Overlays are usually hinged down one side with adhesive tape and, when required, are turned over to lie flat on the projector. They can be mounted so that they can be used in any sequence with the base transparency or they can be added in a fixed sequence so that they will always appear in the same order. The overlays may have to be trimmed very slightly to allow them to fall easily into place.

The illusion of movement—blood flow, for example—can be achieved by using a special attachment that fits over the projector's working surface. This calls for special materials, and relies on the movement of one transparent film relative to another.

Many radiographs can be projected successfully with an overhead projector. The room has to be darkened and as much of the radiograph as possible masked off, so that there are no bright patches of light beyond the area of interest.

Conclusion

The overhead projector is a valuable, versatile visual aid, usually for lectures, but also for small groups. It can be used in a well-lit room with the lecturer facing the audience and completely controlling the presentation. It can also be used to focus discussion in small-group teaching, and to provide information with results in a group problem-solving exercise. It is a good substitute for the blackboard, and with proper use is much more versatile.

Further reading

McRae R K, *The overhead projector*. Medical Education Booklet No 4. Dundee: Association for the Study of Medical Education, 1975.

20 Use slides

Mary Evans

What is conceived well is expressed clearly.
Boileau

The standard of visual presentation of data has improved in recent years, but too many people still show "railway timetables" (fig 1), and the faded bluish purple Diazo slides known disrespectfully as "aged professorial". It would help us all, I think, if somebody invented a way of incorporating a mechanism into slides that caused them to self destruct after two years or so. Pioneers including Calnan and Barabas,[1] and Dudley[2] laid down the principles of clarity, simplicity, and readability 20 years ago, and these still hold good whatever the method of production that you use.

"None can be said to know things well who do not know them in their beginnings"[3]; perhaps people are not taught that slides have three purposes—to give background, evidence, and illustration —and that is why it is necessary to reiterate the principles so often. Slides should be used to put the work being presented into perspective, to summarise the evidence, and to illustrate the results. The correct function of slides is to complement a talk in the same way that pictures enhance an advertisement and "give a truthful, exact, apt and striking description of the goods advertised".[4]

Many lessons may be learned from the world of advertising. Ogilvy wrote that "the purpose of illustration is to telegraph the message to the reader",[4] and a useful rule is that if a slide cannot be understood by the audience in four seconds it is a bad slide; if people have to concentrate on working out the message of a slide they are

ORGANISM	ROUTE OF INFECTION	TRANSMISSION	CLINICAL SIGNS PUPPIES	ADULTS	P.M. FINDINGS IN PUPPIES MACROSCOPIC	MICROSCOPIC	DIAGNOSIS	TREATMENT AND PREVENTION
STREPTOCOCCI (Lancefield groups L and G	?	Bitch to bitch	Only some puppies in the litter fade.	Abortion, Sterility, Cessation of oestrus and Tonsilitis	Enteritis, Degeneration of kidneys and liver Lungs consolidated Subcutaneous oedema.	Cloudy degeneration of liver and kidney	Isolation of organisms P.M. Findings	Chloramphenicol during pregnancy Autogenous vaccines
E.COLI (?Haemolytic)	Oral (vaginal discharge milk)	Dog to bitch	Whole litter fades	Diarrhoea, Genital infection in dogs and sterility.	General congestion, Haemorrhagic gastritis, Oedema of Mesenteric Lymph Nodes	Gastric lesions (Lymphocytic infiltration and submucous haems. Desquamation of epithelium	Isolation of organisms P.M. Findings (gastric lesions)	Streptomycin, Chloramphenicol, Autogenous vaccines, Treatment of stud dogs.
BRUCELLA (?GB)	?	?Dog to bitch	?	Abortion, Genital infection in dogs and sterility	?	?	Isolation	?Streptomycin
TOXOPLASMA	In utero Oral - milk	?	Only some puppies in the litter fade. Some deaths may occur in older puppies.	Abortion, Enteritis, Cough Nervous signs	Muscles pale ? Placenta ?	T.gondii cysts	Serology Isolation Histopathology	Pyrimethamine and Sulphonamides

Fig 1 A typical "railway timetable". Too much information has been badly laid out, with no consideration of proportions or readability, and the whole picture has been more confused with the addition of both vertical and horizontal lines.

not listening to the speaker. Good slides can be shown at the rate of one every 50 seconds.

Slides of text and tables

Slides should not be used as *aides-mémoire*. There are still many (usually inexperienced) speakers who face the screen and declaim the text of each slide to the last syllable; it does not seem to occur to them that if they can read the slide, the chances are that the audience will also be able to.

There are seven adjectives that should describe good text slides: appropriate, accurate, legible, comprehensible, well executed, interesting, and memorable. If any of these (except perhaps the last) cannot be used to describe your slides, scrap them and start again.

Appropriate

Tables, graphs, and drawings produced in enough detail for journals (where they may be studied at leisure) are unsuitable for slides. The salient points should be abstracted and, where possible, presented as pictures, cartoons, or diagrams that produce an immediate effect. If words must be used, then only a précis should be given. Yorke showed the virtue of abbreviation when he pointed out that if Nelson's signal had read "With reference to previous instructions appertaining to naval discipline, it is felt that all personnel in the immediate vicinity of Cape Trafalgar will carry out

118

the navigational and/or combative duties allocated to them, which-ever is applicable, to the satisfaction of all concerned", instead of "England expects that every man will do his duty", it would have been neither obeyed nor remembered.[5]

Accurate

> I do not mind lying but I hate inaccuracy.
> Samuel Butler

It should be unnecessary to make this point. I have, however, seen the following spelling mistakes on slides shown recently at national and international meetings: ileostemy, seperation, assesment, femerofemoral, iliorectal, coexistant, and—one of the most com-mon—anastamosis.

Richard Asher's plea is well founded: "However good your memory is, you should look up everything you quote".[6] One should add "and then check it again". This is particularly true if the slides are being typed by someone who lacks a detailed knowledge of technical terms. Always check artwork for spelling before having it photographed.

Errors are not always accidental, nor are they restricted to text. When drawing a graph, for example, it is possible to show bias to the point of dishonesty if you draw it with a vertical axis showing 40% at the bottom and 45% at the top, instead of 0 at the bottom and 100% at the top.

Legible

The size of a slide is 35 x 22 mm. Whatever you are show-ing—text, diagram, pie chart, histogram, graph—the proportions of 35 to 22 should be strictly adhered to. So if the width is fixed, you should multiply by 22 and divide by 35 to give the correct depth; and if the depth is fixed, you should multiply by 35 and divide by 22 to give the correct width. This ensures that full use is made of the space available. Of course these instructions do not apply if you are using one of the computer-assisted systems for the construction of slides, as the proportions are built into the software.

It is important that only a limited amount of information should appear on each slide. Some of the computer-assisted systems have a word allowance built in, but if you are not using such a system this objective can be achieved by insisting that you do your own artwork.

You will find that it takes much less time to make a simple slide than a complicated one. Too often medical art departments are expected to produce sensible slides from material suitable only for publication. There is no better way to clarify your thoughts than to be obliged to construct the slides yourself. An added advantage to making your own slides in these days of competition and money making in the health service is that many medical art departments now charge for their services. It is easy and cheap to construct your own professional-looking slides with the help of a word-processing package and a camera.

Transfer lettering, such as Letraset, is supplied in sheets, and used to be one of the few ways in which amateurs could give their lettering a professional appearance. It produces excellent work when spacing and alignment are carefully measured, but the process is slow and expensive. As with other methods, the optimum size of type is 24 point on A4 (297 x 210 mm) matt cartridge paper with margins of 30 mm all round. It should be possible to read the original artwork from a distance of four metres.

Several other rules should be observed to achieve legibility. Use bold typeface to obtain maximum clarity. Never use full stops—they disturb the visual flow of type—and use other punctuation marks sparingly. Choose capital letters and lower case consistently. Use capital letters for titles and lower case for text; it is more pleasing to see a line completely in upper case or completely in lower case, except where initial capitals have to be used for proper nouns. People read lower case typescript more quickly and easily than upper case. Eric Partridge quoted from the preface to *Webster's International Dictionary* of 1934: "It should be clear to even the meanest intelligence that the unnecessary use of capitals may easily lead to ambiguity or, at the least, to discomfort and resentment".[7]

Thirdly, use space between letters, words, and lines with care. Research into the design of road signs showed that the largest observed effect on reading distance was produced by changes in spacing (fig 2).[8]

Fourthly, use a sanserif typeface (one without the "tails" on the letters). It is easier to read at a glance,[4] though a serifed face is preferable on the printed page (fig 3). Attractive and legible typefaces are Helvetica, Microgramma, and Univers.

Finally, in a "summary" slide points introduced by asterisks or bullets (dots) are more arresting than those labelled with numerals: 1, 2, 3, and so on. Quite apart from the visual effect, numerals

120

Fig 2 The effect of increasing the space between the letters by 1 mm at a time in each line. In the middle line the optimum spacing has been achieved.

Fig 3 Different sizes of a sanserif typeface (Helvetica), left, and a serif typeface (Century Schoolbook) right. The optimum size on a sheet of A4 paper is 24 point.

121

indicate a diminishing order of importance, which is not always what one wishes to convey.

Comprehensible

How often have you heard a speaker comment apologetically "This slide may look rather complicated." It is usually an under-statement, and signifies only that the speaker has not taken the trouble to simplify it. Two or three simple slides are better than one unreadable one that is crammed with data. Complicated formulas and detailed experimental methods have no place on slides. They need only be mentioned by the speaker, and those who want the details can be referred to published work.

Abbreviations, though tempting, should be used with care—particularly if the audience is international. Standard ones have been published,[9] but it is sensible to keep them to a minimum and explain those that you do use.

Well executed

Though well executed is closely related to "legible", it should be remembered that "an ugly layout suggests an ugly product".[4] Slides should be well balanced and, where possible, designed to be shown horizontally (landscape) rather than vertically (portrait), as there are surprisingly few lecture halls in which the screen does not cut off one end of a vertical slide. Always write horizontally when annotating the vertical axis of a graph. Never under any circumstances do your final drawing on graph paper, as the background lines will confuse and distract.

The choice of the method of photographic reproduction is a matter of taste and opportunity. Large traffic signs (such as directions on motorways) have light-coloured lettering on a dark background,[10] and this principle has not changed with time (fig 4). Dark lettering on a white background is not as easy to read, and such slides have the disadvantage of showing every speck of dirt and dust with which they have come into contact.

Negative slides are the quickest and easiest for the amateur to produce, and colour can help to achieve balance as well as being important in other respects. It can be helpful to have all the headings or references to a particular feature in the same colour, and certain colours have natural associations that can be used to advantage. We are brought up to recognise, for example, that red implies heat or danger; green, safety; and blue, peace or cold. A most useful colour

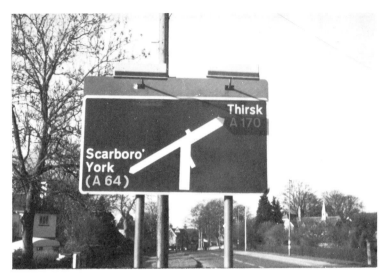

Fig 4 A "primary route" sign showing the sanserif typeface printed in light lettering on a dark ground.

is white, not only in its own right[11] but also to "point" or balance other colours.

If you are making your own negative slides you will need a single-lens reflex camera, Kodalith 35 mm film (and the appropriate developers), and two No 2 Photofloods. The exposure is $\frac{1}{2}$ second at f8. Colouring and mounting should be done together, and require back lighting, which is most simply provided by a portable x-ray screen. Slides need protection, and should be mounted between glass; the grey and white Gepe mounts are ideal (though expensive). Mount the transparency on the grey side and secure it with masking tape. Then apply the colours directly to the face of the film, ideally with Staedtler Lumocolor pens (designed for use with overhead projectors). If you cannot get these, any coloured felt-tipped pen will do (for example, Golden Platignum "painting sticks"), though care should be taken, as sometimes the points are rather thick. Any small flaws in the developing process (which show up as white dots or lines) can be concealed by using black felt-tipped pen or masking tape.

Graphics packages for computers are proliferating, and there are many on the market; they vary in price between a few hundred pounds and several thousand. Most are user friendly only to people

123

who are already familiar with programs like Windows. Good slides can be made with such packages, but I do advise caution. Firstly, most packages have been designed primarily for business presentations, and it is difficult to draw a scattergram or a survival curve. Secondly, by putting an unlimited number of colours at your disposal, they positively encourage lack of restraint. Thirdly, and most importantly, unless you use them often you will not get the best out of them; you will take an inordinately long time to make a simple slide, and this is simply not cost-effective.

My own preference is to marry the most useful of the new technology with the most cost-effective of the old. I have saved a layout in my word-processing package that automatically gives me eight lines of 24-point Helvetica bold italic, and I print this in landscape format on A4 paper on a laser printer. The artwork is then photographed on Kodalith film and I colour the negative slide by hand.

Whichever type of production you choose, you will make a bad impression if your slides are not mounted straight or if they are dirty. Always put an adhesive dot in the bottom left corner of the mount to help the projectionist (there are seven incorrect ways of showing a slide). Check your slides just before handing them in; transparencies can slip within the mounts in transit even when secured by tape. If possible load them into the carousel yourself. Take spare mounts with you in case the glass of a vital slide is broken.

Interesting

"You cannot bore people into buying".[4] If your slides are dull, inaccurate, badly made, and illegible your audience will go to sleep or leave the hall. As Hopkins pointed out, "A person who desires to make an impression must stand out in some way from the masses",[12] and this is particularly important if you are presenting one of 50 or more papers at a research meeting where each speaker has a particular axe to grind.

Some people have tried to make their presentations more interesting by adopting the relatively new technique of dual projection. Beware: it is not an easy technique to master. It should never be used merely to show double the permitted number of slides. It has a limited, but useful place. For example, a courtesy to an audience whose first language is not English is to project at least the most important slides in the language of the host country at the same time

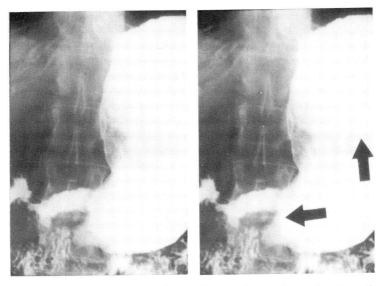

Fig 5 Left, a barium meal examination showing a carcinoma of stomach and a peptic ulcer; right, the same picture but with arrows indicating the lesions.

as showing the slides in English. If you do this, put blank slides (preferably glass mounts with self-adhesive foil on them, as this does not allow the light to show through) in the carousel when there is not a matching English slide so that the two projectors can proceed in tandem. You will have enough to worry about while you are giving the paper without trying to remember which projector should go forward and which should not.

Memorable

There are few memorable slides. We all know which they are—we remember them.

Graphic slides

Coloured slides and halftones should be clear reproductions that show only what you wish to illustrate with as little background "noise" as possible. So that the audience does not waste several seconds looking for the feature that you are showing, indicate it with a self-adhesive arrow (fig 5).

Much useful advice about the design of graphics has been given by

125

Tufte.[13] Among his essential points are that graphs must not lie; the data must be shown; the "data:ink ratio" must be maximised, and all "non-data-ink" and "redundant-data-ink" must be omitted. Data ink is the ink that is used to disclose data, and the data:ink ratio is the ratio of the parts of the graph that disclose data to the total amount of ink used in the graph. Overcrowded slides always irritate (fig 1).

Line drawings should be drawn on matt cartridge paper in thick black ink. Again, if the feature that you want to illustrate is not immediately obvious, indicate it with an arrow.

Graphs, histograms, scattergrams, and pie charts should also be drawn clearly in black on matt cartridge paper. One of the disadvantages of some of the computer graphics packages is that the lines are extremely faint and do not photograph well, so do make sure that if you use such a package you draw over the lines with a thick black pen.

Presentation[14]

Dress formally and not flamboyantly. Keep still and beware of mannerisms in speech or action that might distract or irritate the audience. One of the common faults of even some experienced speakers is to use the light pointer to draw attention to a slide, and then forget to turn it off. This leads to the "mad moth" syndrome as the light darts distractedly (and distractingly) around the hall.

There is rarely a place for jokes in a presentation, particularly on the part of junior members of staff. A witty aphorism is permissible, but it should never be forced.

The ideal speaker does not wander about the platform as if searching for an exit, and does not wave his or her arms or the pointer for emphasis. Rather, this speaker establishes a rapport with the audience by being enthusiastic about the subject and by referring to a previous speaker's comments. The slides will be easy to read from the back row of the hall, and the talk will have a beginning, a middle, and an end.

Speakers who follow all these rules make it look easy, but you can be sure that they have taken a lot of trouble to get the slides correct; they have rehearsed with their slides in front of an audience of colleagues (which is often harder than giving the paper at the meeting); they have probably changed the order of their slides several times; and they have not memorised their talks—there should always be room for spontaneous remarks.

Conclusion

I wish I could say (*pace* Samuel Johnson) that when a man knows he is to speak in a fortnight it concentrates his mind wonderfully. Even more do I wish that this would be reflected in the quality of his presentation.

1 Calnan J, Barabas A. *Speaking at medical meetings*. London: Heinemann Medical, 1972.
2 Dudley H A F. *The presentation of original work in medicine and biology*. Edinburgh: Churchill Livingstone, 1977.
3 Temple Sir William. Preface to History of England. Quoted by: St Arnaud G. *Legislative power of England*. London: Thomas Woodward, 1725.
4 Ogilvy D. *Confessions of an advertising man*. London: Longmans, 1964.
5 Yorke G C. *Working with words*. London: Blackie, 1965.
6 Asher R. *Richard Asher talking sense*. London: Pitman Medical, 1972.
7 Partridge E. *The gentle art of lexicography*. London: Andre Deutsch, 1963.
8 Christie A W, Rutley K S. Relative effectiveness of some letter types designed for use on road traffic signs. *Roads and Road Construction* 1961;**39**:239–44.
9 Biblis M, ed. *Dorland's medical abbreviations*. Philadelphia: W B Saunders, 1992.
10 Moore R L, Christie A W. *Research on traffic signs*. Proceedings of a conference on engineering for traffic. London: Printer Hall, 1963.
11 Chesterton G K. A piece of chalk. In: *Tremendous trifles*. Beaconsfield: Darwin Finlayson, 1968.
12 Hopkins C. *Scientific advertising*. London: McGibbon and Kee, 1968.
13 Tufte E R. *The visual display of quantitative information*. Cheshire, CT: Graphics Press, 1983.
14 Pollock A V, Evans M. The ten-minute talk. In: Troidl H, Spitzer W O, McPeek B, *et al. Principles and practice of research: strategies for surgical investigators*. 2nd ed. New York: Springer-Verlag, 1991: 384–7.

21 Look after a visiting speaker

Patrick Hoyte

In the course of my work for a medical defence organisation I have lectured around 150 times in five years. Some of the audiences have been non-medical—for example, health economists, nurses, administrators—and some have been students, but most of my speaking engagements have been to medical audiences of one sort or another —postgraduate societies, BMA divisions, courses for trainee general practitioners, courses for family planners, specialist symposia.

Anyone accustomed to this sort of regular lecture circuit will be well aware of the immense variety of venue, host, and hospitality. While the venue itself may not be too important, provided one has been given the information to find it at all, some standards of hospitality leave a lot to be desired; although I am happy to say that the really bad examples are very much in the minority.

Two disasters . . .

In February 1988 I was asked to speak to an evening meeting of a medical group in the Midlands. I specifically asked the organiser for a slide projector to be made available and went ahead with travel arrangements, including a hotel booking. When I arrived at the venue after a 60-mile drive, I found that the meeting had been cancelled because there was no projector and that the organiser had sent only a deputy to apologise. Given an audience, I could, of course, have spoken perfectly well without visual aids, but was not consulted, although the cancellation had been announced only earlier the same day. No offer of a lecture fee, travelling, or subsistence expenses was made.

Six months previously I had spoken to a specialist symposium at a major teaching hospital. There was no one to meet me when I arrived, as the organiser was listening to the previous speaker. The promised meal was almost all gone and was in any case cold, and there were no clean plates, cups, or cutlery. The previous speaker exceeded his time by about half an hour, and it was another 20 minutes before the visual aids (in this case a video recorder) could be made to work for my own presentation. Even though it was an evening meeting, no lecture fee or travelling expenses were paid.

. . . and a triumph

The following evening I was contracted to speak to a postgraduate society in Lincolnshire. Maps of the town and of the hospital were sent to me and a parking space was set aside; the organiser and the postgraduate secretary were waiting in the doorway to greet me; I was offered an excellent meal and choice of drinks and placed with pleasant company; I was even shown the "gents" without having to ask. The meeting itself went well, the large audience asked a lot of stimulating questions, and informal discussion went on for some time after that. A lecture fee and travelling expenses were paid and I received a pleasant "thank you" letter from the postgraduate tutor.

Dos and don'ts

The examples I have given are clearly opposite ends of a large spectrum, but I do not doubt that the "disaster" organisers would have been quick to criticise if my presentations had attained only the standards they apparently set for themselves. I therefore put forward the following slightly tongue-in-cheek aide-mémoire for the benefit of those who wish to invite visiting speakers and who want to look after them properly. Needless to say, I have my own blacklist of venues; I hope that some of the organisers concerned will recognise where they themselves have gone wrong.

(1) The initial letter of invitation should give basic information about the requirements and current level of knowledge of the likely audience and set out the format of the proposed meeting: duration of

talk, degree of formality or informality, time allowed for questions, other speakers and their subjects, panel discussion.

(2) The size of the prospective audience should also be given. Speakers are understandably aggrieved if they give up an evening (or indeed any other period of time) and find only a handful of people present. If the attendance is likely to be small and the speaker is told in advance, he or she may well wish to refuse the engagement. My own threshold level is around 20 to 25, but I appreciate that this information is hard to come by and that many organisers are not prepared to commit themselves on this point.

(3) A follow-up letter a week or two before the meeting should include directions to the venue. The correct motorway exit is always useful, together with any inside knowledge about the town's inevitable one-way system. For large hospitals, a map showing the position of the lecture theatre is often necessary. Parking problems should be identified and a temporary permit provided if a formal system operates; no lecturer at the end of a hard evening wants to find that his car has been wheel-clamped!

Speakers should be told if a meal is to be provided (before or after the lecture) or whether they are expected to fend for themselves en route. They should also be told if the catering is in any way idiosyncratic—as a confirmed carnivore I find compulsory nut cutlets pretty depressing and I suppose that vegetarians must have the same problems, although perhaps more often.

(4) On the day the organiser should arrive at the venue before the speaker; it is perhaps surprising how often this does not happen. If the organiser cannot attend, the name of his or her deputy should be sent to the speaker in advance.

(5) Before the start of the meeting the speaker should be introduced informally to a few selected members of the audience so that he or she starts off feeling welcome and in pleasant company. No speaker should be left standing alone in a corner, or with only a drug company representative to talk to. Nor should the speaker be saddled with the postgraduate society's most awkward or paranoid member who everyone else is trying to avoid.

(6) If there is no meal attached to the meeting, the speaker should at least be offered a cup of coffee and perhaps a sandwich before or after his or her performance, or both. The distance travelled may have been considerable and perhaps a meal had to be missed to fit in with the timetable.

The speaker should be given the opportunity to visit the toilet before starting. There is nothing worse than getting half way through a planned lecture and feeling that you should have "gone".

(7) When introducing the speaker, the chairperson should be sure about the correct pronunciation of the surname and should also add a first name. It is profoundly discourteous to introduce "Dr Smith" or worse "Dr J Smith", when a single inquiry would allow "Dr John Smith" to be used. A little bit of background biography is also easy for the chairperson to elicit; it is helpful for an audience to be told something of the speaker's credentials.

(8) The speaker will have indicated what is required in the way of visual aids. The organiser should have checked that these are available and in working order, and should know which buttons operate the equipment and lights in the lecture theatre.

(9) The chairperson should have a couple of prepared questions "up his or her sleeve" in case the discussion period after the formal lecture is slow to get going.

(10) Doctors from within the NHS who lecture "for love" should certainly receive a proper fee and should be told of the amount in advance. The same criteria apply for the reimbursement of travelling and subsistence expenses.

If several doctors appear on the same programme, they should all receive the same fee. Speakers naturally tend to congregate together and it is highly embarrassing for one to find that another is receiving a higher (or lower) fee.

(11) If the meeting has been successful, the organiser should send a brief "thank you" letter. This simple courtesy particularly applies if no fee has been offered, or if a cheque for a relatively small amount will take three months to arrive from an anonymous NHS or university finance department.

(12) Lastly, the organiser should always remember that the speaker will have had to work hard to prepare the lecture and that he or she may well have had to travel a considerable distance to deliver it, at some personal inconvenience, and with the loss of home comforts. The organiser therefore has an obligation to treat the speaker with courtesy and a duty to provide a sizeable, alert, and inquisitive audience.

22 Travel to a conference (obtaining funding)

K C B Tan, D J Betteridge

That first major scientific meeting tends never to be forgotten. Until then, senior, national, and internationally known colleagues are but names on well-thumbed papers and reviews. Suddenly there they all are, in the flesh so to speak, either presenting new data or taking part in the discussion of the work of others. Somehow senior figures (at least most of them) seem to be approachable on these occasions and are readily available to give advice and help with scientific matters.

Of course, the occasion can be daunting and sometimes overwhelming if the young research fellow is to present his or her first paper in front of the leading figures in their subject. Anxious thoughts cross the mind. Have I rehearsed enough? Will I dry up? How does the microphone work? Will I get my slides the wrong way up? Will professor so and so ask difficult questions? and so on. It is much better to have sampled the atmosphere of these large meetings—in some specialties there may be over 5000 delegates—before the fateful day of the first paper.

Later in your career the excitement of these meetings pales slightly through familiarity, but they remain a source of intellectual refreshment and ideas. New friendships are made, old ones are renewed, and mutual problems can be discussed. The benefits of attending national, European, and world congresses in your subject are incalculable, and this is especially true for younger people. But raising the money to get to them may seem to be an impossibility. Money can be particularly tight in the research years because available funds cover only payment of the basic salary with no units of medical time. Some of the larger units will have what are commonly called "slush" funds which can be used for funding travel to meetings; such units are relatively few.

So how do you set about raising the necessary money to cover travel and accommodation expenses? Furthermore, the registration fees for meetings seem to be rising exponentially and may well be over £100 a person for a large international meeting.

Funding from the specialist associations

Most specialist associations set aside money, often from major pharmaceutical companies, for the provision of travel grants to junior members. Age limits vary but are usually below 35 years. It is therefore very important to join the appropriate specialist organisation at an early stage. Their funds are, of course, limited and preference is often given to first and second authors of abstracts that have been accepted for presentation at the meeting. Detailed scrutiny of the advance notices for meetings is required, as applications for assistance towards travel costs often have to be submitted at the same time as the research abstracts. This can be up to nine months before the meeting. If several abstracts are submitted from a single department, some thought as to the order of joint authors can ensure maximum benefit for junior colleagues.

Funding from employers

Travel expenses, subsistence allowances, and registration fees can, in certain circumstances, be obtained from your employer, be it a university, district, or regional health authority, depending on the particular grade of appointment. The overriding principle in negotiating this often tortuous bureaucracy is to plan well in advance. In most cases retrospective claims are not considered. It is not possible to detail here all the regulations concerning study leave and expenses, but enlist the support of your consultant or head of department where appropriate. The postgraduate dean and clinical tutor should point you in the right direction. It is unlikely that junior doctors will receive financial support from health authorities for overseas meetings except in the case of senior registrars presenting their own work. The same restrictions do not apply to university posts, and most universities have funds available for non-tenured staff, although these are strictly limited and often will not cover the full cost of an overseas meeting.

Major grant-awarding institutions

It is worth applying to the major grant-giving bodies such as the Medical Research Council and the Wellcome Foundation with requests for travel grants, especially if you are already funded by them. Bear in mind, however, that the travel grants awarded by these institutions go mainly to support short visits to other research groups for the exchange of ideas or to learn new techniques. Of course, this important activity could appropriately follow on from a scientific meeting overseas. You must apply well in advance for these awards.

Royal colleges

The royal colleges make travel grants available to members and fellows often in the form of named fellowships. These fellowships provide funds for postgraduate activities and research in prestigious overseas departments for varying lengths of time. They are not primarily designed for attendance at scientific meetings, but a scientific meeting could be an important part of the package of activities.

The Royal Society will consider applications for travel grants from postdoctoral fellows and senior doctors in certain circumstances, so it is worth obtaining a copy of their regulations.

Pharmaceutical industry

The industry provides considerable funds for travel to and registration at major national and international meetings. This is often done in association with the local organisers of the particular specialist body and the activity is acknowledged in the conference programme. Some pharmaceutical companies also advertise travel grants in the weekly journals, inviting applications, which are decided on a competitive basis. In both these instances preference is given to those presenting abstracts that have been accepted for presentation at the meeting.

It is a great advantage for research fellows to have attended one of the major meetings before presenting their own work. But it is much more difficult to obtain funding in this instance unless the particular department where the fellow works has funds available. The pharmaceutical industry may be very useful here. Of course, it helps if the research fellow works in an area in which there is a lot of industry interest. In our view this is a legitimate activity, although some will disagree. Make initial approaches through the relevant local representatives, as chances of obtaining funding are often enhanced if the representative is pushing the case. Turn down the offer to discuss this or that product over lunch but tactfully suggest that help towards the travel costs of the next European meeting would be a more worthwhile way to spend the budget.

Make the most of the money raised

Advance programmes for many international scientific meetings provide the facility for booking convenient hotel accommodation beforehand. Furthermore, members of particular speciality associations receive unsolicited details of "package" deals to attend forthcoming major meetings. We have never availed ourselves of these opportunities, believing that good, cheaper alternatives are often possible. This does not apply to national meetings when adequate and cheaper accommodation is to be had in university halls of residence.

The traditional "bucket shops", which deal in the "unsold stocks" of airline tickets, have been heavily criticised because of financial losses and non-arrival of tickets, but some of these outlets are good and efficient: the difficulty lies in knowing which fall into this category. If you want to deliver your talk to your colleagues at the meeting rather than to other stranded passengers at the airport, it is best to use Association of British Travel Agents (ABTA)/ International Airline Transport Association (IATA) bonded travel agents whenever possible.

Planning ahead is the most important consideration in obtaining the best deals. Cheaper excursion flights (stay includes a compulsory Saturday night) have to be booked at least two weeks ahead for most European flights, and three weeks ahead for those further afield. Consider charter flights/accommodation packages, such as city breaks, which can be very good value, especially if you share a room with a colleague. Choosing an unpopular flight time (early morning, late night) may enable cheaper tickets to be obtained. For Europe it is worth considering rail travel, and for a small group travelling together driving may prove much cheaper. We know of some colleagues who actually camped out near one European city and travelled in daily for the meeting. For those not so hardy, there are now plenty of available guides that detail cheap and clean basic accommodation in most cities.

Conclusions

It is well worth the challenge to raise money to attend the major meetings in your relevant specialty. An ex-chief known to us refused to give any of his research fellows financial help to travel. His parsimony led to an excellent training in raising money.

III RESEARCH AND COMMUNICATION

23 Plan a research project

Michael Warren, Robin Dowie

Disciplined inquiry, review of current practice, audit, and research are components of the practice of medicine. Each of these related activities requires detailed planning and the writing of a protocol, which will be the yardstick for the measurement of progress and achievement in the project and may form the basis of an application for a research grant.

The protocol should set out the aims of the project, how these are to be achieved, how bias will be eliminated, the subjects or types of patients to be studied, the ethical aspects, and the proposed statistical and/or other analyses to be used. It should establish that the expenditure of effort, time, and money is likely to be worth while. Statistical, computing and other expert advice should be sought at the preliminary stages of planning.[1]

The questions and suggestions listed below are intended as an *aide-mémoire* for those planning a project, whether this is to be a descriptive study, a clinical trial or a survey.

The protocol

What is the purpose of the project?

What are its aims and precise objectives? What questions is the project intended to answer? Is the purpose to test, examine, or evaluate current practice or a new treatment, procedure, or service, or to obtain new facts about the causation or natural history of a disease?

What is already known about the issues to be investigated?

What are the gaps in present knowledge? How will the proposed project contribute to knowledge and understanding of the problem? What might be the applications in practice of the results of the study? How might these be achieved?

There are a number of centres that can provide information about past and current studies in various fields[2] and, in England, advice can be obtained from the regional directorates of research and development.

Is the proposal for a pilot or a main study?

If a main study is proposed, the details of the pilot study should be included in the proposal.

What design will be used in the project?

Will the project be basically a laboratory study, a clinical trial, or a survey? Will it be a trial of an "intervention"—for example, a treatment, procedure, or service (therapeutic, preventative, caring, or educational)? Will it be a case-control study with randomised or matched controls, or a quasi-experimental study? If a survey, will it be conducted by use of questionnaires, interviews, or clinical examinations? Will the study be retrospective, cross-sectional, or prospective (cohort)? Is a "blind" or "double-blind" design proposed?

How are the subjects of the project to be chosen?

What is the population from which the subjects will be drawn (the denominator in incidence and prevalence studies)? Are the subjects of the project the total population of a community or all patients with a certain diagnosis, impairment, or disability? What are the entry and exclusion criteria for selecting subjects for study? How are the controls to be chosen? Will a sample of the total population or of all potential subjects be used? If so, how is the sample to be obtained to ensure that it is representative of the total group?

The number of subjects (or sample size) must be large enough to allow analysis of multiple factors and to obtain significant results.[3]

What data are to be collected, and why?

What factors (variables) are already thought to affect the outcome? What new factors are being tested in the study? What extraneous factors, if present, might distort the general representativeness of the results? What are the indicators or measures of the outcomes of the trial or experiment?

The amount of data collected should be limited, though measures of different dimensions of outcome should be used when possible.[4]

What are the treatment schedules or other activities forming the "intervention" in the project and how are the variables to be defined and measured?

Have the techniques, dosage, programmes of treatment, prophylaxis, and other activities been standardised? This is especially important in multicentre studies.[5]

Have explicit decisions been taken about how the presence or absence of disease is to be determined (for example, hypertension and diabetes), how duration and severity are to be measured, and how social and demographic variables (for example, marital state, occupation, socioeconomic group, and ethnicity) are to be defined? The proposed definitions and measurements should be consistent, wherever possible, with those used in comparable studies; if this is not possible, the reasons should be stated.

How are the data to be collected and the measurements to be made?

Will the data be collected from records, observations, interviews, or examinations of the subjects? Will special recording forms be needed? Who will collect the data? What training will they need and how will this be arranged? Should an independent observer make the baseline or outcome measurements (or both)? Have the methods been tested? Are they valid: do they actually measure what they are intended to? Are they reliable: can they be repeated to yield the same results? Are they sensitive: can they identify all positive cases? Are they specific: can they identify only positive cases? What checks and controls will be used to maintain accuracy and objectivity during the collection of the data?

How will the data be processed and analysed?

What statistical and computing help is required? What is available? Will any of the data have to be coded? If so, who will do this? Who will do the data entry? How will the analysis proceed? How will the results be presented? What will be the form of the report?

Are there problems of ethics and etiquette associated with the project?

Are patients'/subjects' rights properly protected? How are the consent and collaboration of patients, interviewees, doctors, nurses, social workers, and others to be obtained? How is the confidentiality of the data to be ensured at each stage of the project? What agreements will be made about publication of the data and the report? Has the project been approved by the relevant ethics committee?[6]

What arrangements are to be made for advising or treating people for whom new needs come to light as a result of the project?

Can the local services cope? Have they been advised about the project? Will special arrangements be required?

What is the timetable for the project?

In what order will the different stages of the project be carried out? What is the duration of each stage? Who will be involved at each stage?

Enough time should be allowed for analysing the data and preparing the report; that is, the presentation, synthesis, and interpretation of the raw data.

What will the project cost?

What will be the cost of each stage of the project? What will be the cost in workforce, including the estimated costs of the time of the main investigator, advisers, and others not directly employed for the project? What will be the cost of additional salaries, including pension and national insurance contributions? What will be the cost of the rent for the accommodation for the project? Is capital equipment required? What is the estimated expenditure on travelling and subsistence, stationery, printing, postage, telephone, and photocopying? Are there computing costs? What outside help and advice are needed? What are the administrative costs and overheads? What are the possible costs to the NHS or other organisation involved in the project?

The protocol should state clearly what is already available and what additional resources are required.

Sources of funds

There are a number of sources of funds available for the support of research, including the NHS, the Medical Research Council (MRC) and a wide range of charitable organisations.

The Department of Health has set out its strategy and priorities for research and development in the NHS.[7] The criteria for funding projects are that the project should:

• be designed to provide new knowledge considered necessary to improve the performance of the NHS in enhancing the nation's health;
• be designed so that the findings will be of value to those in the NHS facing similar problems outside the particular locality or context of the project;
• follow a clear, well-defined peer-reviewed protocol approved, where necessary, by the local research ethics committee and any other relevant body;
• have clearly defined arrangements for project management;
• have the clear intention to report the findings so that they are open to critical appraisal and generally accessible.

The Scottish Home and Health Department, Welsh Office, and the Department of Health and Social Services, Northern Ireland, have comparable arrangements for funding research and development.

The main emphasis of MRC-supported work is on biomedical research, although the council now has a health services and public health research board. Other grant-giving bodies range from the large national institutions, such as the Nuffield Provincial Hospitals Trust, the King's Fund, and the Wellcome Trust, to organisations concerned with research into particular diseases and patient groups. Charities that are members of the Association of Medical Research Charities (AMRC) each spend more than £250,000 a year and use peer review in the allocation of grants.[8]

Applicants for research funds may be required to complete a detailed application form. Such a form must be completed fully and in the manner prescribed. Research committees and referees are not impressed by an applicant who has not taken meticulous trouble over the submission and provided realistic estimates of the duration and costs of the proposed project. If an applicant wishes to provide additional information, this should be done on separate sheets and referred to in the appropriate place on the form. The applicant should inquire from the funding body whether there is a particular date by which applications must be received. Some research committees meet annually, some twice a year, and some more often. Some committees like a proposal to be seen by referees before it comes to the committee, while other committees screen all proposals before seeking expert advice. Either way, to miss a meeting can delay the start of a project by many months.

1 Useful introductory references are Abramson J H. *Survey methods in community medicine*, 4th ed. London: Churchill Livingstone, 1990; Altman D G. *Practical statistics for medical research*. London: Chapman and Hall, 1991; Cartwright A. *Health surveys in practice and potential: a critical review of their scope and methods*. London: King's Fund, 1983; and Pocock S J. *Clinical trials: a practical approach*. Chichester and New York: John Wiley, 1991.
2 The Department of Health has established a Project Registers Coordinating Unit in Harpenden, Hertfordshire, and a Centre for Reviews and Dissemination in York. Other sources of information are the Cochrane Centre at Oxford concerned with randomised control trials and other reliable data about health care, the specialist centres and units funded by the Department of Health and the Medical Research Council, and the UK Clearing House for Information on the Assessment of Health Outcomes at Leeds.
3 For guidance on sampling and sample size, see Abramson (1990) and Altman (1991) in 1 above.
4 See Long A F. The outcomes agenda: contribution of the UK clearing house on health outcomes. *Quality in Health Care* 1993; 2: 49–52; Fitzpatrick R. Surveys of patient satisfaction I and II. *BMJ* 1991; 302: 887–9 and 1129–32; Fitzpatrick R, Fletcher A, Gore S, *et al*. Quality of life measures in health care I, II and III. *BMJ* 1992; 305: 1074–77, 1145–48 and 1205–9; and, Drummond M F and Davies L. Economic analysis alongside clinical trials. *Int J Tech Assess Health Care* 1991; 7: 561–73.
5 Cancer Research Campaign Working Party: Trials and tribulations: thoughts on the organisation of multicentre clinical trials. *BMJ* 1980; 281: 918–20.
6 See Medical Research Council: *Responsibility in the use of personal medical information for research*. London: MRC, 1985; Medical Research Council, *Responsibility in investigations on human participants and material and on personal information*. London: MRC, 1992; and Department of Health, *Local Research Ethics Committees*. London: Department of Health, 1991.
7 Department of Health, *Research for health*. London: Department of Health, 1993.
8 See Association of Medical Research Charities. *Handbook 1993–4*. London: AMRC, 1993; and Charities Aid Foundation. *Directory of grant-making trusts 1993*, 13th ed. Tonbridge: CAF, 1993.

24 Organise a multicentre trial

C Warlow

Multicentre and single-centre clinical trials share methodological problems which are well known (see box). Multicentre trials do, however, have several distinct advantages. They provide:

- larger sample size so that the result is more precise, appropriate subgroup analysis is more feasible, and there is a lower risk of an apparently "negative" result when the treatment is, in truth, effective;
- quicker results before people lose scientific or commercial interest in the treatment, and before it is modified or the theoretical basis for it is changed;
- wider dissemination of the results and, possibly, more widespread belief in their validity as well;
- standardised definitions of disease and measurements of outcome among centres and also among countries in international trials;
- a wider range of clinical and methodological expertise to solve protocol problems;
- usually a wider range of patients, facilitating the generalisation of results that can be broadly applied to future patients in other centres and other countries;
- large "negative" trials, which are more likely to be published than small "negative" trials. This is important; otherwise, small "positive" trials, which are more likely to be submitted for publication and probably more likely to be accepted than small "negative" trials, will tend to dominate the scientific literature and so lead to publication bias;

Methodological issues common to both single and multicentre trials

- Randomised or non-randomised treatment comparison
- Blind or open treatment allocation and outcome assessment
- Intention to treat, or on-treatment analysis, or both
- Sample size and duration of follow up
- Subgroup analysis
- Defined entry and exclusion criteria
- Amount of data to collect on randomised and non-randomised but eligible patients
- Defined outcomes
- Widespread applicability of trial results; what to do about non-randomised but eligible patients
- Interim analysis and the role of an independent data monitoring committee
- How intensively to monitor compliance
- Computerisation of data
- Sharing of original data with overview groups looking at similar treatments (meta-analysis)
- Involvement with sponsoring company, if any.

- less suspicion and rivalry among centres and countries without necessarily suppressing healthy competition;
- less scientific isolation;
- better national and international collaboration;
- facilitation of further multicentre trials of potentially important treatments, provided the initial trial is not too exhausting.

The difficulties of multicentre trials compared with single-centre trials mainly concern the coordination of many people in several centres and even countries. The issues that may present particular difficulties are:

- leadership
- writing the protocol
- finding the centres
- randomisation
- patient registration
- follow up
- trial coordinator
- trial office
- visiting the centres
- collaborators' meetings
- quality control
- cost
- writing the papers.

There are usually several possible solutions, the best depending on circumstances, geography, number of centres, the budget, and so on. What follows is not meant to be an ossified blueprint but some suggestions—suggestions, moreover, that have not been tested in randomised trials but that, at least, are based on some experience.

Leadership

A multicentre trial must have an identifiable leader or principal investigator, who should be able to command the respect of collaborators and have the time and energy to keep the whole enterprise under control. He or she must not lose interest in the dull bit between getting started and getting the results. Running a trial by committee is disastrous. A prestigious chairperson of a steering committee may be a "political" advantage, or even a necessity, but such a person is unlikely to run the trial on a day-to-day basis. Someone must get the funding, gather together centres, run meetings, answer questions, solve problems, visit centres, and set up and supervise the trial office. This person will usually, but not always, be a doctor, presumably whoever wanted to set up the trial in the first place, and someone who is going to be in the same job long enough to see the trial through to the end. A medically qualified principal investigator must try to enter his or her own patients in the trial to maintain credibility, and to experience and share the practical problems with the other collaborators.

Writing the protocol

Writing the protocol is a job for one person, usually the principal investigator, and not a committee. Of course, that person will need comments and advice from all the centres, the trial statistician, and outside experts in the field, and this may require one or more collaborators' meetings and often several versions of the protocol before everyone is satisfied. Because there is no rule against modifying a protocol if unforeseen problems arise during the trial (provided such modifications are sensible and not dependent on data analysis), there is no reason to delay writing it and getting started while some centres finally make up their minds whether to join in. Indeed, it may be desirable to involve more centres once the trial is under way and some of the teething problems sorted out, although the more centres that are involved from the very start the better. It does not always hold, however, that centres involved in writing the

147

protocol are more likely to stick to it than centres joining later and having to accept it. In international trials the protocol may have to be translated into several languages, which can be surprisingly expensive. Fortunately, if it is written in English, translation is now hardly necessary, at least not in Europe, which is a huge advantage to us in Great Britain and a great credit to our medical colleagues on the continent.

Finding the centres

Having accepted that a multicentre rather than a single-centre trial is scientifically necessary to solve a particular treatment problem, friends and colleagues from a few centres usually get together to discuss a protocol. From there, other friends and colleagues are brought in from centre to centre, and from country to country until enough centres are found to satisfy the sample size requirements in a reasonable period of time. After about three years recruitment gets tedious and may fall off, but follow up is usually less time consuming and may need to continue much longer, depending on the treatment. Key people in a country are often very successful in recruiting their own compatriots, far more so than an outsider. Advertising in medical journals and through specialist organisations can also help. Pharmaceutical companies may, through their national and international networks, approach numerous potential collaborators simultaneously.

However the centres are found, they must be seriously interested and reasonably competent in the field, but not necessarily specialists. In any event specialists may already be involved in their own competing studies; relative non-specialists in district general hospitals or general practice may be extremely keen to collaborate—and make very effective collaborators. Usually they have more patients than teaching hospitals, they may have no other way to take part in medical research, or to be involved with specialists in the field who are organising the trial which is often educative. But whoever the collaborators are, they are all equal when it comes to recruiting patients and it is *their* trial, not the principal investigator's (whose role is organisational and catalytic); there should be no "star billing".

Randomisation

Randomisation must be centralised and is best done by telephone, or perhaps by a computer link, to some central point, which may be the trial office or, if 24-hour cover is required, a hospital ward or switchboard. This is the only way for the trial organisers to have an immediate binding record of who has been randomised, when, and from which centre. Sealed envelopes or locally held randomisation lists are simply not good enough.

Patient registration

If large numbers are required and the budget is limited, patient registration must be simple, practical, and quick. Collaborators should have to do little more than what is normally required in routine clinical practice. Patients must be identified (name, sex, date of birth), data on a few important prognostic variables collected, and possible prespecified subgroups identified. It is often feasible to collect all or some of these data on the telephone before treatment allocation is made, so obviating the need to complete, post, check, code, and punch data entry forms. It also means that the treatment allocation is not made unless and until the entry data are recorded centrally. Another advantage is that data recorded *before* randomisation are unbiased with respect to any knowledge of treatment allocation. Computer networks that perform the same function are another possibility, but more expensive.

Superfluous data must not be collected and nor should "add on" studies be allowed without adequate human and financial resources. Indeed, all the collaborators must have a very clear idea of the aim of the trial and concentrate on that. Nevertheless, it may be possible for a few particularly interested collaborators to collect more data than the others, but this should be optional and certainly not to the detriment of patient recruitment or answering the basic trial question.

Follow up

Follow up must also be simple and require little more than would be done in routine clinical practice. Obviously, the outcome must be recorded and measured, but this may not require frequent follow up, and sometimes it can be obtained from routinely collected data (such as death certificates, cancer registries, and so on), thus disposing with the need for patient follow up at all. Some follow up might be more simply, and even more accurately, obtained by telephoning or writing to the patient or carer rather than by contacting the patient's doctor. Overelaborate recording of and testing compliance should be avoided, as should unnecessary blood tests. Too frequent and too detailed follow up may add very little to the statistical power and may kill recruitment in a multicentre trial once trial contributors realise what they have let themselves in for. Written forms should be no longer than one side of A4 paper; if they are, they probably will not be completed fully or reliably. In any event trials should not interfere with routine clinical practice.

Trial coordinator

The trial coordinator is the key person even if the trial is not large enough to merit a full-time appointment. The job is administrative, not medical. She, for it is seldom he, stands at the centre of the trial and must be committed, energetic, sensible, well organised, have some knowledge of computing, and be able to work flexible hours. To collect the data, organise them, and transmit them to the statistician, she must be meticulous and even obsessional, but she must also be good with people so that she can run the trial office and maintain harmonious relationships with the distant collaborators. She must be adroit at dealing with the awkward (and some doctors can be remarkably awkward), and flexible and energetic enough so that she can hop on and off trains and planes and put up with a certain amount of discomfort as she travels from centre to centre extracting data from forgetful collaborators, encouraging them to randomise more patients, and generally nurturing *esprit de corps*, while still retaining a sense of humour.

Trial office

The trial office, organised and supervised by the trial coordinator, has the task of collecting, checking, and entering the data from the distant centres and requesting more information if there are inconsistencies or omissions. The office must supply the collaborators with all the necessary documentation (entry and follow up forms, freepost envelopes, sticky labels, and so on) and possibly even the trial medication; dispatch regular newsletters and listings on missing data and listings of when patients are due for their next follow up; and answer questions from the many centres. The office must be available, friendly, helpful, knowledgeable, reliable and efficient, perhaps in more than one language for international trials; although doctors may speak excellent English, the same does not necessarily apply to their hospital telephonists. The collaborators must see the office as a "black box" into which data go and out of which information comes. Any strife, inefficiency, or chaos should remain hidden. Such an office needs to be close to the principal investigator and, if possible, to the trial statistician, although with the availability of modern high speed computer links this may not be so important now. The office requires secretarial and clerical staff, a telephone and answering machine independent of a busy hospital or university switchboard, a fax machine, a photocopier, several microcomputers, printers, filing cabinets and adequate storage space. It must have enough resources to do its job properly and take as much as possible of the burden of the trial organisation from the collaborators. The resources required will gradually increase through the recruitment period, after which they will stabilise, but probably not decline.

Visiting the centres

Visiting the centres is time consuming and expensive but may have to be done, often regularly in order to:

- discuss any local problems arising from understanding and implementing the protocol;
- encourage recruitment to the trial and solve problems relating to this;
- collect outstanding data, although with advance warning these usually appear in the trial office shortly before the visit;
- discover neighbouring centres interested in joining the trial;
- reinforce the role of each centre without which the trial would fail;
- keep everyone informed of what is going on in the trial as a whole.

The meeting must be arranged well in advance because it is important to get *all* the local collaborators around a table. But the visit need not last long, perhaps an hour or so. Remember, the local collaborators are busy and the trial is unlikely to be their major preoccupation or priority. Who does the visits depends on the circumstances; the trial coordinator is usually the best person to collect data, and the principal investigator is best at sorting out scientific and medical problems, but a regional coordinator can be helpful if the centres are widely dispersed. Whoever it is must not waste time; several centres can often be visited in a day and work can

151

be done on trains. Trains with sleeping compartments allow an early start to the day to be made. Avoid visits during the summer, when collaborators are on holiday and the trains are full of additional passengers, and avoid the depths of winter when snow and fog dislocate transport. Don't carry too much with you but take enough to read in case you get delayed; take train and plane timetables and be prepared to change your plans; sort out how to get money quickly in foreign countries; don't forget a telephone charge card; and make sure the trial office and your family know your whereabouts. In very large trials visiting each centre is impractical, but regional meetings of several centres is an alternative.

Collaborators' meetings

Meetings of collaborators are needed to write, and if necessary, rewrite the protocol; to discuss disease definitions, measurements of outcome, and documentation; to discuss any interim results; to encourage recruitment; to plan new trials; and to encourage a group identity and common purpose. They are, however, time consuming to attend, extremely time consuming to organise, and expensive. They should therefore be frequent enough to fulfil their purpose, but not so frequent as to be prohibitively expensive. It may be sensible—or even essential—to organise regional or national collaborators' meetings if there are a large number of widely dispersed centres. It may also be possible to link trial meetings to others that collaborators are likely to be going to anyway, such as national specialist societies, international meetings, and so on. Furthermore, it may be scientifically attractive (and indeed commercially attractive if registration fees and sponsorship are forthcoming) to organise a symposium or educational meeting alongside the trial meeting.

Quality control

In a single centre trial it is important that the trial treatment is properly described, well delivered, and any complications fairly assessed. This is even more important in multicentre trials where there are certain to be differences among centres, both real and due to chance. Even trial drug treatment may differ because of different storage conditions or possibly circumstances of delivering it to the patients. But of more concern is variation among centres in non-drug treatments being evaluated, such as surgery, speech therapy, psychotherapy, and so on. Obviously all the centres must agree more or less to standardise such treatments so that about the same amount is given, for about the same time, and that it is reasonably uniform. Such non-drug treatments, however, will never be *exactly* the same in all centres and it is counterproductive to insist that they are; as long as they are roughly similar no problems will arise and the trial result will be applicable to other centres giving roughly, but never *exactly*, the same treatment. Monitoring uniformity of treatment is difficult but at least it helps to monitor any immediate complications, such as postoperative morbidity. If a centre is performing badly (inadequate treatment, excessive complications, not enough patients to ensure competence, and so on), then it should stop randomising patients, but not, of course, stop following up those already randomised. Clinically sensible cointerventions, such as drug regimens administered during a trial of a surgical procedure, do not have to be exactly the same in each centre because randomisation (stratified by centre if necessary) will ensure that they are used in the same proportion of "treated" and "control" patients across the trial participants. In a multicentre trial there may be more strenuous efforts made than in a single-centre trial to ensure that the treatment (both trial and cointervention) is properly delivered and discussed, so that generalising the results may actually be more appropriate; in a single-centre trial the treatment programme may be less likely to be submitted to peer review, criticism, and audit.

Cost

Multicentre trials are expensive but they need not be prohibitively so provided the collaborators are reasonable and do not attempt to re-equip their entire department and undertake major non-trial projects at the expense of a sponsoring pharmaceutical company. Indeed, from the point of view of unit cost per patient randomised, or per patient year of follow up, multicentre trials should be cheaper than single-centre trials, as they gain from economies of scale. But, of course, the trial office and collaborators' meetings must be properly funded, and the collaborators themselves reimbursed for any extra work (which is very little in a well-designed trial) over and above routine clinical practice. There are various ways of doing this: a lump sum for every patient randomised; a sum for every completed data form received by the trial office; a formula based on the number of patients randomised to support a research nurse, and so on.

Whatever is decided, the collaborators should be paid only for extra work done, and not work that they say they will do. In many trials, however, it is very difficult to obtain proper funding. This applies particularly to treatments from which no profits are to be made—for example, non-patented drugs, surgery, physiotherapy—so that it is totally inappropriate for all trial funding to be left entirely to the pharmaceutical industry. Although a sponsoring company must not be involved in either data analysis or publication, it can be extremely helpful in collecting baseline (but *not* outcome) data, maintaining trial discipline, and encouraging recruitment through its own networks of medical representatives and researchers.

Whatever the cost of a trial, it should be compared with the incidence, prevalence, and cost of the disease being treated and, perhaps, against the cost of non-medical endeavours, such as low-altitude military aircraft training or unemployment benefit. By any such comparisons, multicentre trials are usually extremely inexpensive and may lead to the rejection of expensive but ineffective treatments—for example, extracranial to intracranial bypass surgery for the prevention of stroke—and not always to the introduction of more expensive health care.

Writing the papers

Like the protocol, writing the papers is a job for the principal investigator, not a committee. Naturally, it will be necessary to have many discussions with the trial statistician and trial coordinator, and comments and advice from all the collaborators, as numerous drafts are produced. It is crucial that in the end all the results are published under the names of all the collaborators: without them there would have been no trial at all and they did the work. Although unfashionable in some quarters, the whole philosophy underlying multicentre trials is that group effort takes precedence over individual effort; only by acting as a group can the individuals get answers to therapeutic questions that affect their own individual patients. Of course, any centre can publish its *own* results, but there must be no "star billing" for authors when the results of the whole trial are presented.

Conclusions

Before starting a multicentre trial the following questions must be answered affirmatively:

- Is the therapeutic question really important, preferably even a burning issue?
- Are you sure there is no better way of answering it?
- Can you get enough centres together?
- Are you likely to get the resources?
- Have you got the time?
- Do you *really* want to do it?

If so, then go ahead, but first visit one or two successful multicentre trial organisations, which will give you far more idea of the problems and pleasures than I have been able to within the context of this article. Remember, only fools fail to learn from others' mistakes. And once you get started, always keep thinking about how the trial can be done more efficiently and effectively, less expensively, more quickly with a greater recruitment rate and with less extra work being done by the collaborators. At the same time, remember that *esprit de corps* is what counts more than anything else: look after it.

25 Chair a conference

Ronald Gibson

Although much depends on the type of conference—the size, the length, the subject—certain basic principles are common to all.

Firstly, I think it is vital that you have some idea why you have been elected to take the chair. It may be because of age or experience, a reputation for being a good chairperson or—and this is well worth remembering—because successive efforts to find someone else have failed. You might have been low on the list when the conference was first mooted. It is a salutary thought that you have been the first sucker to accept.

Being elected to the chair by the conference itself has its advantages. It is usually the culmination of years of effort on your part or it may be quite unexpected; in either case, you can reckon to have at least a nodding acquaintance with most of the members. The disadvantage is that you may find when you sit in the special chair reserved for the chairperson that it isn't a bit like you thought. Suddenly you are alone and isolated from the rest of the conference. Friendly faces previously surrounding you on the floor can now be seen only at a distance. They look nothing like as friendly from your new seat (or is this your imagination?).

Have you, you wonder, a friend in the hall? This may be the first time that you experience that oft to be repeated temptation to cut and run. Resist it. Have a quick look round from your throne as you sit waiting for the clock to tell you it is time to start and make a note of those you see (preferably scattered about the hall) who could form the nucleus of a reliable MI5 for you. This is particularly helpful if the conference lasts more than one day.

156

However long it lasts, you must expect the sense of isolation to persist; even the buzz of conversation round the bar or in the dining room will suddenly dry up as you arrive to take some much needed refreshment. This may be due partly to respect and (which is much more likely) partly to the traditional but unwritten rule that the chairperson must not be party to any opinions they may be expressing or plots they may be hatching.

The individual behind the bar (who has extraordinarily acute hearing), the ushers, or even the hall porter can often, unwittingly, be members of your MI5 ("Good morning, chairman, I hear they've got it in for you today" is well worth the conversation about the weather you shared with him or her the night before).

In spite of your sense of isolation, however, it is unwise for you not to seem to be mixing with the members during the conference. They like to have a close look at you and to feel that, in spite of the possibly irreparable damage they are doing to your health, you are still one of them and they tend to resent seeing you only at a distance. You cannot afford to be aloof or incommunicado off stage. There is always hanging over you the threat of "no confidence in the chair". You are less likely to be faced with this if you display obvious regret that it is impossible for you to talk individually to each member of the conference (though this is what you would like to do and may actually feel you've done by the time the conference ends). Do not forget, also, to exhibit commendable humility throughout.

Helpers and others

The first friend you must make is the secretary of the conference: he or she is steeped in a subject of which you have only superficial knowledge, and without his approval and advice your tenure as chairperson can be constantly at risk. Establish a happy working partnership from your first meeting (which should be well before the conference opens). Ask to be briefed on the subjects to be debated and possible snags. Ensure that you are informed of any particular characteristics of the conference—each usually has its own. Those taking part have personality traits, foibles, paranoias, and motivations that are peculiar to their trade and which it is unwise to disregard. When you know the secretary well enough, gently try to prise from him or her some personal knowledge of those taking part. This is a delicate subject, but it is always wise to have a list of those capable of making life difficult for you and of others who can be relied on to get you out of trouble: the humorists who may try to take the mick out of the chair (they can turn out to be your best friends), and those who although—in your view—full of sound and fury signifying nothing, must be treated with the greatest respect (if slighted they can be your worst enemies).

Having established a happy working relationship with the secretary (at the same time paying due compliments to his or her clerk or personal assistant) and given tacit assurance of your implicit obedience, next turn your attention to bylaws and standing orders. These are usually inexplicable hell, and it is as well early on to persuade members that you are congenitally incapable of interpreting them. This brings you down to their level without them having to confess their own ignorance. It also has the additional advantage of ensuring that they are on your side when you are challenged by the inevitable member who knows standing orders by heart.

Rigid adherence to standing orders and an inability to stretch them if the conference so wills is unwise. On the other hand, there are two that the chairperson must know: the procedure to be adopted on the motions either that "the question be now put", or that the conference should now "pass to the next business". Any hesitation from the chair after these suggestions may lose the confidence of members. It is sometimes possible, indeed desirable, for the chair to anticipate these motions by hinting to a sympathetic member (through a third party) that, by one or other of the available alternatives, a particular debate should be closed—it is as well that some subjects should not reach voting stage and that others should not be overdebated. I believe that at such times it is the chairperson's duty and, indeed, prerogative, to sense the feeling of the conference and help members to disentangle themselves before any permanent damage is done.

Preconference homework having been done, the chairperson will take the chair with apprehension, tachycardia, and loss of nerve. These feelings are necessary if the conference is to be successful, and they should in no way be distorted by taking alcohol or tranquillisers. Yet, of course, they must be disguised from the members: the chairperson must present an appearance of calm and fortitude.

The human touch

When opening the conference I suggest that you address the members briefly. You should emphasise that you are, of course, their servant; your object is to develop a happy family atmosphere; you will do your best (you say) to be absolutely impartial and ensure that every speaker gets a full hearing. You add, somewhat regretfully, that they will understand you are merely human and bound to make mistakes, for which you can only throw yourself on their mercy. You then show that you have a sense of humour by including a little throw-away quip, and end up by intimating that, despite your acknowledged inadequacies in the chair, you can exhibit a punch like a kangaroo if necessary. This latter comment must, of course, be put over by inference or innuendo and accompanied by a bland and innocent smile, yet there must be no doubt that it is clearly understood.

The conference will then, with luck, proceed peacefully—at any rate for the first hour or two. You must be benign and generous, fixing the members with an occasional smile, which they will come to know means you think they are being good and are proud to be their chairperson or, on the contrary, that you think they are being very clever but they had better "watch it" before they go too far. This is very different from setting out to control the conference from the word go. I have seen a chairperson determinedly stand up to members in the mistaken belief that, by so doing, he was proving that he was the boss. In fact he was oppressing opinion and antagonising delegates.

With the help of your friend, the secretary, you will soon get to know who are the clowns of the conference and who the potential chair destroyers. Let the first have their way until you sense the conference has had enough. Let the latter have plenty of rein until they think they are about to deliver the *coup de grâce*, and then give a tug calculated to pull the bit through their mouth and halfway down their throat. The timing requires careful calculation because members are watching the battle, they know the rules of the game and will not tolerate any infringement; they don't want it to end before they have seen two or three rounds, yet they will not forgive the chair if its opponents triumph (nor will the opponents strangely, they too are aware of the challenge and are prepared to yield to a manifestly better person).

Although a gentle quip from the chair directed toward the speaker is not a bad thing, it must be seen to have a friendly intention. Members don't enjoy the chair being funny or clever at the speaker's expense, but will happily accept a little amicable fun, even though they know there may be a tiny bite attached to it. It is far more likely that members will support the chair (with which they may secretly be in agreement) if they are allowed to set a speaker down themselves; there is nothing to be gained by the chair trying to do this job for them and thus run the risk of switching sympathy over to the speaker.

War and peace

So you will proceed. Peacefully and unobtrusively guiding the debates but never failing to be attentive. Strangely, it may be that you will not take in a word that is being said. This is all right—subconsciously you are keeping one step ahead and you are relying here on the secretary to nudge you if you appear to have missed a vital point. Try to avoid being in communication with an eager member who wants to fire a question at you from over your shoulder—arrange for someone to accept and note such questions and pass them on to you, if he must, between debates.

The more peaceful the proceedings (if you are wise) the more concentrated your attention, for round the corner may be the crisis that besets all conferences at least once. It is what I call the "gadarene swine motion". Often it is initiated by a comparatively unknown, young and enthusiastic member speaking to what at first seems to be an innocent and inoffensive motion. The little fire he or she lights is fanned by successive speakers. Suddenly there is an ominous silence in the hall; the secretary sharpens a pencil (with luck, he or she warns "this is it"); others on the platform start to fidget; a queue of speakers forms at the microphone; the press is agog, for the conference is about to exhibit its authority over the Establishment, of which you are part. You are on your own and you will never have felt so lonely. Any attempt to limit the length of speeches or the number of speakers will be noisily resisted. Any show of dissent by the Establishment will be howled down. Members are enjoying themselves—so at last, is the press. Let it go. Do not entertain suggestions that you pass to the next business or that a vote be now taken. You must play this one and it may take an hour or more. Never lose your grip, yet never be seen to enforce your authority. Hope that the very force of the flames will put the fire out before it is too late. I have never found it productive to try to appeal to the good nature of members—on these occasions they haven't any. Far better to wait for them to play themselves out, then—when the acute phase is over—it may be possible to extricate the conference from the results of its orgy before a vote is taken. More than this you cannot do.

After this, purged and passive, contrite members—suddenly realising what they have done—will be clay in your hands. With pained (but not angry) demeanour you may now lead them through twice or three times more motions than normal. This, together with a soporific after-lunch session, is of immense value to you in speeding through the business of the conference. The suffering you have endured will have been worth while.

Getting through the remaining important items of the agenda now has priority. Before the penitent reaction is over it can be productively used in getting members' permission to pick special items out for debate, putting others aside for discussion later (if there is time). They will almost certainly approve, howling down any dissenters as part of the redemptive process. Although each member will regard his or her particular motion as of the utmost importance—it is not for you to disabuse anyone—you must be ruthless in overriding some. Your objective is to finish the day with major decisions having been taken and the *raison d'être* of the conference substantiated. Once you have done this to your satisfaction you may attend to the rest of the agenda, knowing that even if you don't debate every item, the conference has effectively produced an informed opinion.

At the end, some kind soul (primed to do so by the secretary if you have not by now offended the latter beyond words) will propose a vote of thanks to the chair. You will be duly applauded by all and sundry—including, you hope, the press—who, although they have appeared to make life hell for you over the past few hours, have really been your good friends and welcome this opportunity to show their devotion.

Now is the time for the double whisky (repeated, if desired) and it is surprising how quickly the pulse rate returns to normal.

I am more than conscious of my failings as a chairperson, yet I am fairly certain that they would have been fewer had I been able to stick to the guidelines I have so glibly suggested here.

26 Organise an international medical meeting

Ian Capperauld, A I S MacPherson

Committees and budgets

At some time in their professional careers doctors may be concerned with organising a medical meeting. Meetings range from large international ones to small local gatherings, but the principles for organising all of them are the same. We propose to state these principles, to expand on topics that are often alien to the medical mind, and to point out some of the pitfalls that may trap the unwary and uninitiated. The principles are simple, and some of the things we say will seem obvious, but the obvious is often overlooked merely because it is simple. We shall discuss committees, budgets, scientific and social programmes, registration, and other aspects of medical meetings.

The framework

Committees

The organising committee must be carefully chosen by the chairperson. This working group of people will have various tasks allotted to them, many of which will be time consuming. It is important, therefore, to allot duties to suitable individual members. It would be disastrous to assign a task that demands a frequent presence to a member of the committee who flies round the world every week. Similarly, you should think carefully about giving some jobs to the young who have energy, and others to the mature who have tact. Each member of the organising committee should chair a subcommittee to coordinate the main activities.

An important point in choosing the organising committee or some of the subcommittee members is to include lay people. Obtaining the help of someone in local government will smooth the path to official receptions, while the city manager or one of his or her senior colleagues on the committee will produce facilities and services that are invaluable to the meeting. Similarly, including a lay member who knows about finance and budgeting is imperative. If a trade exhibition is to be held, the help of someone in the pharmaceutical industry will keep that side of the meeting under control and add to the income. The chairperson should appoint subcommittees for the following (with a member of the organising committee in charge): scientific programme; social programme; finance and budgeting; audiovisual aids; spouses' programme; publicity, advertising, and trade exhibition; and transport and hotel accommodation.

The organising committee should give a definite remit to the subcommittees, which should report to the main organising committee formally at the main monthly meeting. It is perhaps obvious, but minutes of all these meetings should be kept, and outstanding actions and promises not carried out rectified immediately by the chairperson. Your organising committee should be like the board of a company, whose sole business is to run a successful meeting, ideally at a profit—but certainly not at a loss.

Budgets

Many doctors take fright at the words "finance" and "budget". These aspects, however, are becoming more and more important for a successful meeting, especially as costs rise. Our object is not to tell you how to raise money or what to do with it, but rather to guide you towards good management of your financial affairs. When faced with a medical meeting you must ask yourselves "can we afford it?" and, if the answer is yes, "How can we organise the financial resources to make the meeting excellent?"

The money side of a meeting should be regarded in the same way that you look at your household accounts. You know how much the goods are in the shops and you know how much money you have to spend. By wise buying and shopping around you get value for money. You, in fact, work out the household budget.

A budget is simply a plan of action expressed in financial terms. Essentially, the budget should state how much money is going to be spent and how much money is going to be brought in. Indeed, such an exercise can produce only three results: the meeting will make a profit, will break even, or will incur a loss. Judicial surgical intervention—making certain cuts in the budget—can convert a loss to a break-even, or a break-even to a profit. The first responsibility of any committee is to construct a budget since all other aspects of the meeting are dependent on this.

Cash in

The various sources of money at a medical meeting are direct registration fees, donations, and surplus money from the trade exhibition. Of these, only direct registration fees are completely under the control of the organising committee. Charge too much and you will dissuade many from attending. Charge too little and you may incur a loss. To be certain of viability, therefore, at least 60% of your total income should come from this source. How can you forecast how many people will attend the meeting? Past records help, together with national or current international financial climates. It is important to remember that what may appear to be an excessively high registration fee for someone in Britain may be average or even cheap for someone abroad. In many countries registration fees are tax deductible by medical personnel attending the meeting, and this should be considered when calculating registration fees. The proportion of overseas to home delegates, therefore, could influence the setting of the registration fee.

Donations may be classified as coming from internal or external sources. Internal sources are the cash reserves of the initiating society, and local university and college sources. External sources consist of local government support from city or town councils, and perhaps even central government if the meeting merits such funding. Donations may also come from local industry, which may or may not be allied to medicine, and from industry allied to the theme of the meeting, perhaps even from abroad. You should remember that donations in kind can be just as useful as a monetary donation. Providing a reception, for example, relieves the committee and the participants of cash transfers. Also important in saving money is a waiving of fees for the hire of a building or a lecture theatre.

The income from a well-organised trade exhibition can contribute substantially to a successful meeting, and we give details of its organisation below. Participation by the drug industry, however, requires the courtesy of attendance by the delegates at some time during the course of the meeting, and this is not always arranged. It is a paradox that as more demands are made on the pharmaceutical industry to give support, fewer and fewer delegates appear to be attending exhibitions.

Cash out

Services, buildings, people, and commodities have to be paid for. The expenditure side of the cash budget is readily controllable. The committee can set the amount of money that it is prepared to spend on certain parts of the meeting. A simple example is the entertainment laid on for the delegates. The committee may decide to be lavish or austere. Nevertheless, when the budget is complete, the sum put in for entertainment may be increased to make thrifty entertainment pleasurable, to make lavish entertainment allowable —or legal.

The budget illustrated in the table is taken from an article[1] describing the financial aspects of a large international meeting, and lists the income and expenditure of that meeting. The figure obtained from that particular meeting for registration fees came to 65% of the total income; there was a surplus, or profit, of 16.7%.

Calculations

Responsibility for constructing the budget is a whole committee effort. Every member or chairperson of a subcommittee group should be able to forecast the money needed at least for their own part of the scheme. Start with the list of sums that you will have to pay out. Remember that costs in a budget may be fixed or variable. Fixed means that, whether one person or a hundred turn up, the amount to be spent for that service is the same. Good examples of fixed costs are the hire of the lecture theatre, the projectionist's fee, translation facilities, telephone installation, and insurance. Variable costs depend on the number of people attending and include such things as meals, entertainment, and certain printing costs. It is extremely difficult to be dogmatic in describing fixed and variable costs because some services contain an element of both. Nevertheless, if you stick to the principle of thinking in terms of fixed and variable costs you will avoid the trap of preparing a budget where most of the expenditure is committed to fixed costs.

Having obtained the first estimate of expenditure on the budget, increase this figure by 10–15% to take into account the inflation that

165

is likely to occur between the planning and date of the meeting. Also forecast the number of people who will attend. Given that at least 60% of your income will come from registration fees you can work this out thus:

$$\text{Registration fee} = \frac{\text{total cost} + 10\%}{\text{No attending}} \times \frac{60}{100}$$

If the figure obtained is astronomical you will have to look again at the expenditure side of the budget and cut it until you reach a tolerable level for the registration fee. If such a figure cannot be decided early on, the financial aspect of the meeting spells disaster. Remember that the figures supplied are only guestimates, and the sooner accurate estimates are obtained the better the budget will be. Indeed, the decision of "go" or "no-go" in a meeting can be worked out rapidly by using this formula. When a registration fee has been fixed for years you should be able to obtain an indication of viability by changing the figures in the given formula.

With regard to the income side of the budget, the forecasted number of people attending needs to be accurate to calculate what, in effect, is 60% of your total income. You can relieve this headache by fixing the number of people allowed to attend; this simplifies the budget considerably but does not always lead to a successful meeting. If the attendance is not fixed the income from 100% attendance on as accurate a forecast as possible can be calculated. Similarly, the income from 90% and 80% attendance can be calculated, hence giving you some idea of the money available, which should be balanced by making cuts on the expenditure side. In the early stages the budget should be fluid and capable of being chopped and changed until a definite plan of action is decided. The final income and expenditure statement after the meeting should only confirm the budget. It should be like an x-ray film confirming a previously clinically diagnosed condition.

As we have said, repeated revision of the budget is necessary. It should be brought up to date monthly by the full committee, so that any disasters that are beginning to show up are avoided, or at least ameliorated. The weekly meeting allows pruning of the expenditure if income is not up to forecast or adding a refinement to the programme if the income is above budget. Allowances must be made for insurance in case the meeting has to be cancelled because of airline strikes, hotel strikes, or natural disasters that could affect the

Income	£	Expenditure	£
Registration fees:		Salaries	15.6
Members and temporary		Office equipment	0.8
members	54.2	Telephones	1.4
Guests of members.. ..	10.8	Postage and freight	1.0
Trade exhibition	23.2	Stationery	0.8
Donations	0.4	Insurances	0.9
Banquet	8.2	Expenses of setting up regis-	
Bank interest	1.9	tration offices.	1.3
Advertising	1.2	Expenses of setting up special	
Sundry income	0.1	office	0.4
		Staff travel	0.3
		Sundry expenses	0.4
		Input VAT not recovered ..	0.9
		Sign printing	0.9
		Printing in total.	9.0
		Translation	16.6
		Rents and services	6.8
		Trade exhibition	6.2
		Briefcases and badges ..	0.8
		Transport for delegates ..	0.8
		Banquet	7.6
		Ladies' social club	0.7
		Audit fee	0.8
		Entertainment..	2.2
		Commemorative envelopes ..	0.3
		VIP expenses	2.0
		Hotel bookings not taken up .	4.8
Total	100.0	Total	83.3
		Surplus or profit	16.7

Fig 1 The budget

meeting. The committee should be prepared to pay up to 1% of the total cost of the meeting to get such cover.

One way money may be lost is in misunderstanding whose travel expenses and whose hotel bills are going to be paid by the meeting. The committee should define these invited guests, and include their expenses in the budget. Beware of invited guests who always have caviar and champagne for breakfast and charge it on their hotel bill. Unexpected bills are always sent in—for example, the florist has to be paid for flower arrangements at the official opening and at the banquet. Someone may decide that microphones at the banquet would be useful, and forget that this has to be paid for. Buses ordered and not used have to be paid for, as have staff who stay on because a function overruns. Telephone accounts may come in long after the meeting and often more telephones are laid on or used than have been allowed for. Beware of the individual who asks to use the official telephone and who speaks for half-an-hour at a time with New York, Tokyo, or Sydney, without reversing the charges. Often a guaranteed income is given on bar and coffee takings, and, if this is not achieved, it will be necessary to make up that deficit to the vendor.

In meetings in the UK "value added tax" (VAT) is a problem that should be handled by the accountant. Certain items are subject to VAT and may be reclaimed, while sometimes VAT is payable but not reclaimable. Even corporation tax may rear its ugly head in certain circumstances. When the committee has to be concerned with VAT and corporation tax, professional help is necessary. When the time comes to pay bills, especially when they are large, you should ask whether a discount is available if you settle these accounts quickly.

Trade exhibition

When organising a conference, an important question for the committee must be whether or not to have a trade exhibition. The two main benefits are, firstly, that it can be a useful source of money to add to the budget income and, secondly, that delegates can apprise themselves of a wide range of information about many different products in a convenient and speedy way. Communication with the company representatives can solve problems and queries. If you decide to have a trade exhibition, certain conditions are essential for success:

(1) Committee and delegates alike must acknowledge its value and relevance by according courtesy and attention to the exhibiters and their displays. This is easily done by going to the exhibition daily.
(2) The exhibition space should be an integral part of the conference area, immediately adjacent to the lecture theatre, seminar rooms, or both, and large enough for its purpose.
(3) Morning coffee and afternoon tea, at least, and preferably lunch as well must be served in the exhibition area, which normally should also have registration facilities.

The organisation of the trade exhibition may be handed over to a company whose professional business it is to run exhibitions, in which case the "profit" from the exhibition will accrue largely to that company; or the committee may invite one of the exhibiting companies to organise the exhibition on behalf of the conference, for which only the expenses of the organiser will be charged and hence a bigger "profit" will go to the meeting.

To decide who is to run an exhibition, the committee must consider both the objectives of the conference and its scale. You will find it is a considerable advantage to make the exhibition organiser an *ex officio* member of the conference committee, because this encourages closer liaison and friendly working partnership.

After making the appointment, the committee should agree estimated financial figures with the organiser. These will include such factors as the number of exhibiters who may be safely accommodated in the space available for the exhibition, and also the charge for a square metre of exhibition space. The committee should also, if possible, provide the organiser with lists of potential exhibiters to be invited. Beyond that, they should allow the organiser complete autonomy, subject to periodical reports on progress at meetings of the committee (hence the advantage of his or her membership).

It is well to remember that a conference of any kind is a business occasion and all associated arrangements, including those for the trade exhibition, must be conducted in a business-like manner. While the exhibition organiser will deal with detailed arrangements, the committee should be aware of the main matters to be taken care of. These may be summarised as follows.

Space available

This will determine the number of stands that can safely be accommodated. Adequate gangways to allow stands to be seen and to meet fire safety regulations are also necessary.

Costs

Costs incurred in mounting an exhibition are the rental of space, hire of furnishings and equipment, installation of temporary electricity supply, electricity, and cleaning. These direct costs must be adequately covered by exhibition charges. In addition, participating companies will have their own costs covering stands, publications, samples, travel, accommodation, and salaries. The charge to the exhibiters, therefore, must be carefully worked out so that the direct costs do not exceed the total income from the sale of the exhibition space.

Timing

People staffing exhibition stands will spend the greater part of any day hanging about. It is vital, therefore, to ensure that the length of time the exhibition is on display is related closely to the nature of the conference and the number of delegates. Far better to have a two-day exposure in the middle of a week's conference, than to expect exhibiters to stand around for days on end without a customer. One must also remember to allow time for setting up and dismantling.

Exhibition area

Access for stands and equipment for display must be practical. Electricity supply must be adequate. Water supply and drainage may be necessary. Storage space for exhibiters' material before, during and after an exhibition is essential. Security measures are often required so that valuable equipment is not stolen or broken.

Exhibition organiser

The organiser must be given authority to do the job—and be left to do it. All matters relating to the exhibition must be channelled through the organiser, who will collect and pay out all exhibition money, handing over at the end of the operation a net sum with an audited statement of income and expenditure, with the hope of producing a reasonable profit to the meeting to offset some of the outgoing expenditure.

Conclusion

The problems of running a large international meeting are legion and here we have attempted to outline only some of the main financial aspects. The keys to success are accurate forecasting and tight budget control, coupled with a good accountant and a hard-working committee, meeting frequently, led by an understanding chairperson. The final income and expenditure statement should only confirm the budget previously made. No one should be surprised, therefore, at the profit—or the loss.

Scientific programme

Responsibility for arranging the scientific programme should be given to one member of the organising committee, with powers to appoint a programme subcommittee. Each member of this subcommittee must accept a specific job. The task of the scientific programme subcommittee includes preparing the programme before the meetings, administration during the meeting, and making the necessary arrangements for publication, if this is desired, after the meeting.

Preparation

The topic or topics for discussion must be determined at least twelve months before the date of the meeting, and potential participants must be notified at that time. This is part of the organisation of the whole meeting, not of the scientific programme. If there is a central theme, and the scientific programme is essentially a symposium, the scope and structure must be decided at this time, and speakers and their subjects selected. The invitation to take part should indicate the intended role of the contributors in the symposium, the duration of their talks, and the subjects covered by the speakers on either side of them. In this way, trespass, duplication, and omission are minimised. Written acceptance of the invitation to speak is essential, and its receipt must be acknowledged by the convener of the scientific committee. If translation has been arranged, you should ask invited contributors to send their full typescript to you at least one week before the meeting to allow translators the opportunity of familiarising themselves with the style, content, and terminology.

The programme of most scientific meetings allows considerable time for papers submitted by contributors on subjects of their own choosing, but usually allied to the main theme. One of the first tasks of a programme subcommittee is to send out an announcement that short papers (generally lasting 10 minutes) will be included in the programme, and to invite members to submit or sponsor the submission of summaries. If there are to be poster or film and video sessions this should be notified at the same time, with the request that intending exhibiters should indicate the size and length of the film or tape and the type of tape. You should prepare a timetable for dealing with the summaries, including the following:

(1) The last date on which a summary will be accepted for consideration: to some extent this depends on the size and duration of the meeting, but there are other considerations, which are dealt with below, and, in general, this date should not be later than two months before the final day for registration for the meeting.

NAME OF MEETING AND DATES
Title of abstract in capital letters
Author's designation (Prof/Dr/Mr/Mrs/Ms) . . . . Initials and name (underlined) . . . . Name of town or city. . . . .
The text of the abstract. This should not exceed 250 words.   Please use electric typewriter if possible.

Fig 2 Standard form for summaries

(2) Decision on how many papers can be accepted: this depends on the time available, and 15 minutes, in practice, should be allowed for a paper of about 10 minutes, so that there is time left for discussion.
(3) Arrangement for the scrutiny and selection of papers: responsibility for this may be given to a selection committee of three or four people—the smaller the better—who must report to the committee convener within two weeks. This procedure is made easier if summaries are submitted in triplicate on a standard form that is divided into three blocks (fig 2). The uppermost block is for the title of the paper, the next for the contributors' names and for the place where the work has been done, and the lowest and largest for the summary of the intended contribution, limited to 150 or 200 words. You should already have agreed with your printer the best size for the standard form, and the estimated cost of reproducing the summaries in a booklet that can conveniently be carried at the conference.
(4) Notification of acceptance or rejection: this must be done at least two weeks before the final day for registration because nowadays, unfortunately, university authorities may allow expenses to a meeting for junior staff (in particular) only when a paper is being read. In an international meeting where translation is necessary it is also important to be able to give the translators a chance to look at the summaries, as these are the only indication they may receive of the content of short papers.
(5) Printing and distributing programmes: the completed pro-

gramme should be in the hands of all participants ten days before the meeting, which means being in the post at least four or five days before that.

(6) Reproduction of summaries: the advantage of a standard size and form of summary is that it can be cheaply reproduced by photolithography. The disadvantage is that such a book of summaries is usually too big to fit conveniently into a pocket and has to be carried in a folder. Summaries should be distributed with other written matter at the time of registration at the congress. Sending by post beforehand is unnecessarily expensive.

Recording and proceedings

The decision whether a more permanent and fuller record than the summaries is desirable must be made early in the preparations for the meeting. If it is decided to do so, a willing publisher must be sought and a contract entered into with it. The method of recording must also be decided. Broadly speaking there are two ways of doing this. The simpler, but generally less reliable way is to ask contributors to hand in their typescripts to a designated person at a designated place in the meeting hall at the time the paper is given. This designated person would probably be the selected editor of the proceedings, and contributors must understand that he or she has the usual editor's powers to accept, select, or reject. The second way, which is easier at the time, is to tape-record the proceedings. The advantage of this method is that it also records the discussion. The disadvantage, however, is that the spoken word always has to be extensively edited to make it readable, grammatical, and comprehensible.

If the decision is made to tape-record, it is better to give the job to a commercial firm, which will make all the necessary arrangements for recording and for the first transcription. Illustrations normally have to be ruthlessly pruned, for many more are required to point a moral in a talk than to adorn the printed word. If possible, verbal agreement should be reached between editor and contributor at the time of the meeting on the minimum illustrations necessary for clarity.

Organisation during the meeting

Slides

Wrong slides, upside down slides, out of order slides induce more frustration and profanity than any other feature in a meeting and can easily be avoided. One local member should be in charge of slide collection, arrangement, and onward transmission to the projectionist. A slide collection point should be at a prominent place in the foyer and be conspicuously labelled. It is best to have sufficient slide carriages available for all contributors to be given one. In this they arrange their own slides. The carriage is then labelled with the contributor's name and the programme number of his or her paper and is taken by messenger to the projectionist. In this way all errors and omissions become the responsibility of the contributor. Films and videos should be dealt with at the same collection point, labelled, and then passed to the projectionist. Precise instructions are given to the speaker as to the controls of microphone, lights, pointer and change of slide mechanics.

Chairpersons

Moderators of sessions will have been chosen earlier and must have been clearly briefed on their duties, the most important of which is to keep the meeting moving to time. Each chairperson must know how to work the platform lights and microphones, and be able to pass the information quickly to speakers. Usually, some means of warning speakers that they are approaching the end of their time is installed. It should be as simple as possible, and preferably noiseless —at least until the final ejection stage.

Discussion

In any large meeting the voices of questioners from the body of the hall will need amplification to be audible to both the speaker and the audience. This may be included in the contract for the halls, but should be checked beforehand, and arrangements made for messengers to carry the portable microphones to where they are required.

Registration and its problems

Registration is central to the organisation of any conference and, along with the budget, forms the framework around which the conference is constructed and the timetable devised. It is an exercise in production management, a straight line along which a vast array of details, events, and people have to be programmed. The design of a system of registration is an excellent opportunity for any organising committee to think their project through to the end and, as such, is worth not a little calm and careful thought.

First stages

Ideally, preparation for a large international conference should start two years before the event, and throughout this chapter the timing of the various stages of preparation will be given in the number of months away from the opening date.

Organising secretary

A large conference requires an organising secretary, who needs a permanent office and staff. On a 2-year time scale, the organising secretary should ideally be engaged at 24 months, and certainly by the 18-month mark at the very latest. He or she is in charge of the conference secretariat, in sole charge of registration, and responsible to the local organising committee chairperson alone. The organising secretary services all local organising committee meetings, liaises closely with the chairperson of all subcommittees, and must be kept informed on all aspects of the conference. Policy is decided by the local organising committee and executed by the organising secretary and committee members. Minutes must be kept, listing the duties assigned to the committee members concerned. The organising secretary does not have a vote at committee meetings.

Communication of the conference's requirements to the "outside world" is the most important single function of the organising secretary and, in this respect, we cannot emphasise sufficiently the value of paying a personal visit to everyone whose services will be needed to make the meeting a success. This is especially so with lay people on the committee. In the early days time will be available for this purpose, and it will ease the path towards the final stages when more and more has to be done by telephone. The secretariat will need its own headed paper and telephone number.

The secretarial duties described here assume that the organisation of accommodation—whether in hotels or in university halls of residence—and the allocation of tour tickets are the responsibility of a travel agent, in which case the secretariat need only hold a record of delegates' requirements.

The office

The conference office should be as near as possible to the site of the conference. In the closing few weeks there is an infinite variety of

175

reasons why it is convenient to be near the scene of the final preparations. The office must be large enough to house at least small meetings—say, six people attending—and to store various consignments of conference literature.

The staff

A personal secretary who has knowledge of a foreign language is a boon, especially when multilingual delegates are expected. All outgoing correspondence, however, may safely be conducted in English. At nine months an assistant should be engaged on a morning-only basis to deal with bookkeeping and registration records, and at three months a part-time typist should join the ranks of the secretariat. Efficient and interested staff are the greatest asset to this kind of project. It is astonishing how many details of those attending can be absorbed by interested staff, so that by the time the conference actually takes place you have a hard core of registration personnel with considerable background knowledge.

Accommodation

Having estimated the number of people likely to attend your conference, you must next reserve the accommodation required for the actual meeting in the form of lecture theatres, reception, exhibition halls, temporary offices, and committee rooms. Rooms in hotels and university halls of residence are the remit of the appointed travel agent. Accommodation requirements can often be met by drawing on the resources of your local university, hospital or municipal offices. Do bear in mind that their facilities are often booked years in advance and that you must act quickly. (See also VIPs and invited speakers.)

Publicity

Progress along the line of conference preparation will be annotated by what you choose to make known of yourselves and at what time. Not uncommonly, conference committees produce written information in three stages: the preliminary circular at 18 months; the preliminary programme at 12 months; and the final programme to be collected by delegates on registration. The preliminary circular, in our experience, is unnecessary, since it includes nothing that cannot be contained in a fuller and more satisfying form in the preliminary programme (and it causes unnecessary expense and effort).

Announcements could be placed at 18 months in the relevant

professional journals and newsletters, and a mailing list kept at the secretariat of those wanting further details. As a general note on publicity, do not overlook the usual human capacity to misread and misinterpret information, which will be aggravated when not all the recipients speak English as their first language. Instructions must therefore be brief and clear. The problems and expense associated with providing translation facilities are dealt with below and it may well be that, as a committee, you decide against providing this service. None the less, it is worth producing information on your social programme at the preliminary programme stage in both French and another language.

Distribution

International societies tend to distribute their publications by way of chapter secretaries, to whom circulars and programmes are sent in bulk. Make quite sure that you have the correct name and address of the person concerned and that you are sent notification of receipt. Busy professional people have more to do than write letters, so send them a receipt that they or their secretaries may simply sign and return. If these receipts are not forthcoming within three weeks of dispatch, make inquiries. The chapter secretary, if left undisturbed, may very well make no contact with the local organising committee until it is much too late.

Official carrier

An official carrier should be appointed. In return for a free advertisement in conference publications and representation in your registration area, an airline, usually local, will often provide complimentary tickets for use by committee members on conference business and possibly some of your VIPs, as well as free transport of those bulk packages to your various chapter secretaries. Several airlines will approach you in the early stages of setting up your conference. Whichever one you select should state in writing what benefits they offer as official carriers and what they expect in return. Do not forget that these are details that will have to make printing deadlines.

Preliminary programme

The preliminary programme is a major statement of intent: it states who is meeting, when, where, why, and how. The following are details that it must contain:

Official languages

These are often English, French, and Spanish. By "official" is meant that a paper may be presented in any of the languages mentioned. Nevertheless, it does not guarantee that simultaneous translation facilities will be provided.

Scientific programme

A provisional timetable and list of subjects must be provided along with an application form for contributions. Some important decisions must now be taken—for example:

- the deadline for contributions;
- whether abstracts of papers are to be available during the conference;
- the time allotted to each speaker;
- if there are both symposia and short-paper sessions, do you process the papers differently?

If both symposia and short-paper sessions are to be held, then a book of abstracts is prepared of the latter. Preparing the book of abstracts is made much easier by designing an application form to go with a paper.

The vexed question of translation keeps cropping up. In practice the "simultaneous" translators prefer to have a preview of the paper to be presented. It is impossible to receive all the full texts in advance—even for symposia papers only about half of the texts requested are usually received. In these circumstances translators often have to work from no preparation other than a look at some of the other papers on the same topic. Obviously, for short papers the relevant abstracts are the only preparation material available.

You will almost certainly have to limit translation facilities. The choice lies between keeping the translators together in one lecture theatre or in using their services in different locations during plenary sessions or symposia.

At 24 months you must produce a list of VIPs. Registrations should be checked against this list at regular intervals and VIP documentation marked accordingly. First-class accommodation is earmarked for all VIPs and here, a dire word of warning. As a committee, *you* will have made these reservations; as a committee *you* will be liable to pay for it if the accommodation is not claimed. Make quite sure, therefore, that your VIPs know of your arrangements and that they let you know their firm intentions, in writing by 2 months at the very latest.

Categories of membership

Members usually fall into three groups: full members, who may take part in all proceedings of the conference, scientific, technical, and social; associate members, who are introduced by full members and may take part in scientific and technical parts of the conference, and in the social events if space and numbers permit; family members, who accompany full and associate members and may take part in social events only.

Registration and payment of fees

In the preliminary programme the cost of the various categories of membership should be stated and a penalty date, six months from the conference, on which fees are increased by an amount agreed by the local organising committee. The necessary registration form (fig 3), a printed envelope, and instructions that payment should be made by bank transfer to the organising secretary of the conference should also be enclosed.

Cancellation of registration

The local organising committee should agree a sliding scale of refund and set the dates on which they apply.

Reservation of accommodation

Details of how to apply for accommodation (fig 4) along with a brief description of the various categories available and an approximate price should be stated in full. Make it clear that no reservations of accommodation will be made until the registration fee has been paid. Since accommodation is to be arranged by an official conference travel agent, it is wise to state that the secretariat cannot undertake to make hotel or student residence reservations. Requests for accommodation will inevitably be made to the secretariat, but these must simply be acknowledged and passed on to the travel agent.

General information

The preliminary programme must also contain the following invaluable information: names and addresses of official conference travel agents, carrier, and bank; officers of the society concerned,

(For office use only)	Reg No

Important: before completing this form, read carefully the instructions on page x of the preliminary programme.

Full membership

Surname . . . . Initials . . . .

Title (Prof/Dr/Mr/Mrs/Ms) . . . . Country . . . .

Mailing address . . . .

. . . .

Family members

(1) . . . .

(2) . . . .

(3) . . . .

(4) . . . .

Associate members

Surname . . . . Initials . . . .

Title . . . . Country . . . .

Mailing Address . . . .

. . . .

Registration Fees

☐   Full members at £A (£A + £B if registering after . . . . . .) =

☐   Full members at £C . . . . =

☐   Associate members at £D   =

I enclose cheque/bank transfer No . . . . to cover =
the total cost of my registration fees
and, where applicable, banquet ticket(s)   =

Total   £

Fig 3 Registration form (A4)

including chapter secretaries; local committee members and address of secretariat office; full details of the social programme—however trying it may be to have these particulars arranged one year in advance. Social events include the opening ceremony, trade exhibition, cocktail party receptions, the banquet, and tours of the city and local countryside. (Details of the social programme given later.)

Invited speakers

A word of warning on the subject of invited speakers. Not

Name . . . .

Title . . . .

Mailing Address . . . .

. . . .

Hotels: Grade A hotel—superior first class
        Grade B hotel—first class
        Grade C hotel—second class

Number and type of room required

Grade . . . . Single Room with/without bath

Grade . . . . Double Room with/without bath

Date of arrival . . . .   Date of departure . . . .

University halls of residence . . . .

Number and type of rooms required . . . .
                        Single Rooms
                        Double Rooms

Date of arrival . . . .   Date of departure . . . .

Deposit—instructions, if any, regarding payment of non-returnable deposit

Fig 4 Accommodation Application Form (A4)

surprisingly, many people will assume that as an invited speaker they need not register in advance or pay a fee, and that their accommodation will automatically be reserved on their behalf. Be quite clear as to the scope of your "invitation" and keep a list of invited speakers. It is necessary even for them to process their registration and to apply for accommodation.

VIPs

We had wanted to say more about the mechanics of registration before mentioning VIPs, but the logical time to bring them in is with this note on invited speakers. VIPs are important, and they do have a right to expect that things will be done for them. Nevertheless, as one or two among perhaps 2000 delegates, their interest is best served if, like everyone else, they too complete the official documentation and go through the one and only mill.

Summary

In summary, at 12 months your preliminary programme is dispatched, accompanied by a registration form and application forms for accommodation, social events, and scientific contribu-

181

Reg No	Name	Country	Membership			Fees paid
			Full	Associate	Family	

Fig 5 Sample page of log book

tions, along with a printed reply envelope to be used for everything except the scientific contribution (which is forwarded to the local chapter secretary). The different forms are printed in different colours for easy identification, and for an international meeting the social events, if nothing else, are described in both French and English.

The mechanics

The first completed application forms and registration fees will start to arrive nine months before the opening date. Do not be disappointed by a slow start. The secretariat must count the heads, collect the fees, and keep the following basic records, all of which stem from the information requested in the documentation sent out with the preliminary programme. It is essential that fees be collected by the local secretariat: do not be tempted by an overseas treasure to do otherwise.

Basic records in the office

Each application to attend the conference is registered in a log book, which is written up daily (fig 5).

The log book gives a day-to-day record of the number of delegates attending in any of the various categories. It also gives the name and registration number of the delegate. The registration number is recorded on the registration form, the accommodation form, the social events application form, and on the acknowledgment card, which are all sent to the delegate. Despite the advantages of computer, this manual log book is invaluable.

Registration Card

The registration form is awkward to handle compared with a card, and for this and other reasons the information it carries is immediately transferred to a record card (fig 6), which is kept in a firm transparent plastic envelope and filed alphabetically according to

Full/associate member			Reg No
Surname	Initial	Title	Country
Family members (1) . . . . (2) . . . . (3) . . . . (4) . . . . Total			
Address for correspondence	Conference address in town		
Accommodation requested Yes/No	Hotel/residence No of beds Arriving Departing		

Fig 6 Specimen registration card (actual size 30cm × 13cm)

country. On the reverse of the card should be stated the title of the participant's talk together with the time, date, and place of the meeting. The original registration form now becomes redundant, although we suggest that you do not throw it out.

Social events application forms

Social events applications are also noted in a simple log book. A loose-leaf folder with a section for each event is best. Once again, a day-by-day note is kept of the numbers applying for each event. Once logged, the social events application, along with the requisite tickets (printed in advance), are filed in the same plastic envelope as the delegate's record card.

Accommodation forms

The delegate's registration number is written on the top right-

---

Event . . . . Date. . . . . No of tickets
required . . . .
Banquet (£X per single ticket). . . . .
Date . . . . Signature. . . . .

Fig 7 Social events form (on reverse side of registration form)

hand corner of the accommodation form, which is sent to the conference travel agent after the details of the accommodation requested have been noted on the appropriate record card. Using registration numbers eases communication between yourself and your travel agent in identifying delegates. Complications may arise over foreign names, and you may have delegates with the same or similar names. Tickets and accommodation must be allotted strictly on a first-come, first-served basis, and numbers are a simple guide to precedence. In due course the travel agent will tell the secretariat where each delegate is staying, and this information will also be noted on the record card.

There are three reasons not to have accommodation forms sent direct to the travel agent:

(1) you must insert the registration number,
(2) It is easier for delegates to post one preprinted envelope to you containing all their particulars,
(3) It enables you to keep your records complete and fully up to date.

Let the travel agent bill delegates directly for their accommodation. Delegates do not always apply in time to get the accommodation of their first choice, and a single account from your agent absolves you from making refunds.

Acknowledgment card

After an application to attend has been logged and placed on a record card *and you have received all fees due*, an acknowledgment card is sent to the delegate (fig 8). Delegates must bring this with them as their congress registration card, against which they may complete their registration on site by claiming their congress briefcase. Please note that it is just as important to confirm to delegates that they have not requested accommodation as it is to confirm that they have.

The registration area itself should now be considered and also those expressions of your administrative effort, the conference briefcase and final programme. This section will be completed by a brief summary of the procedures outlined.

Briefcases

Stage one with briefcases is to obtain them and, with this in mind, you may safely start looking for a sponsor at 24 months. Briefcases

```
┌─────────────────────────────────────────────────────────────┐
│                  CONGRESS REGISTRATION CARD                   │
│                                                               │
│  Dear Sir/Madam,                                              │
│                                                               │
│     The organising secretary has pleasure in acknowledging    │
│  receipt of your forms of application and registration fee    │
│  and notes that you do/do not wish accommodation to be        │
│  reserved in City X on your behalf.                           │
│                                                               │
│  ┌──────────┬──────────┬──────────┬──────────┐               │
│  │   Name   │ Initials │ Country  │  Reg No  │               │
│  │          │          │          │          │               │
│  │ . . . . .│ . . . . .│ . . . . .│ . . . . .│               │
│  └──────────┴──────────┴──────────┴──────────┘               │
│                                                               │
│  Please present this card at the registration bureau when     │
│  you arrive in City X.                                        │
│  Secretariat address and telephone number                     │
│                                                               │
│  . . . . . . . . . . . . . . . . . . . . . . . . . . . . . .  │
└─────────────────────────────────────────────────────────────┘
```

Fig 8 Specimen registration acknowledgment card (postcard size)

should be robust and will contain the following: final programme; book of scientific abstracts (unless these are to be sold separately); map and general information on city/country, including a list of restaurants classified according to cost, bus map and timetable; advertising material from sponsoring drug companies; and list of participants.

Social events tickets

Remember that tickets for the various social events have over the months been filed with the individual record cards in plastic envelopes, all stored in alphabetical order according to country. Ten days before the conference you must produce a list of those attending. Obviously, its preparation should be delayed as long as possible, but ten days from the start should be your absolute limit.

Now is the time to take all the social events tickets and transfer them into envelopes, on which is then written the delegate's name, registration number and country. These envelopes are kept aside in alphabetical order according to country at the appropriate registration desk, so that on presentation by delegates of the card acknowledging their registration and fee (congress registration card) two things are handed to them: the envelope containing their tickets for social events where applicable, a stick-on name badge, already completed (which is to be affixed to the briefcase), and a pin-on

185

identification badge, and a briefcase containing all the information needed for all full and associate members.

For the staff, therefore, registration is a question of being handed a card, of going through a file of envelopes, and of reaching for a briefcase from a pile of identically filled cases. It should take less than one minute for a delegate to register and be less complicated than buying a railway ticket.

Proof of registration

The delegate's congress registration card is retained by the secretariat and filed along with the record card as proof of registration. This is not as futile as it may seem: delegates frequently wish to check if their friends and colleagues have arrived.

Registration during the congress

For many conferences the registration area has to be improvised and is normally constructed from a lecture theatre. A typical size for this would be about 60m × 25m. There should be space along one side of the registration area for five registration booths, each the length of two average-sized tables. You could allocate, say, 57 countries to these booths, grouping them loosely according to language and taking care to share the volume of traffic more or less equally. The following are the five registration groups we have found most useful:

(1) Argentina, Brazil, Cuba, Guatemala, Mexico, Portugal, Spain, Uruguay, Venezuela;
(2) Belgium, Egypt, France, Iran, Iraq, Italy, Lebanon, Morocco, Saudi Arabia, Tunisia;
(3) Austria, Denmark, Finland, Germany, Hungary, Netherlands, Norway, Surinam, Sweden, Switzerland;
(4) Australia, Canada, Eire, Ghana, Hong Kong, India, Malaysia, Malta, New Zealand, Nigeria, South Africa, Togo, United States, Zimbabwe;
(5) Bulgaria, China, the Czech Republic, Slovakia, Greece, Israel, Iceland, Japan, Poland, Romania, Russia, Turkey, United Kingdom, the former Yugoslavia.

Also within the registration area must be the conference bank, post office, travel bureau, information desk, refreshments, and seats and tables for use by delegates. Lastly, the secretariat—complete with extra typing staff for the occasion, photocopying facilities, and files and records moved specially from your permanent office.

It is vital that no delays occur at registration. Delegates arrive tired and wish to sign on with minimum fuss. To avoid queues at the registration booths, all queries should be referred to the secretariat. Any delegate who is unable to produce a congress registration card should be escorted personally to the secretariat, where the problem should be resolved. Common causes of a problem are usually a lost card (in which case a duplicate may be issued), or registration fees that have been paid late, in which case no card would have been issued. It is not unusual for delegates from Eastern Europe to prefer to pay on arrival.

Queries may also arise over tickets for the various social events and here you reap the benefit of being able to produce, from the same plastic envelope as the record card, the delegate's original ticket application form.

A cashier is essential in the registration area to handle registrations, including day registrations and ticket payments. Life is much simpler if only *one* person handles cash and if that person has proper facilities.

Throughout the conference, and especially during peak registration times, members of the local organising committee should be constantly on hand to deal with contingencies and to introduce themselves to any delegate who looks lost. The impression this gives, and justifiably so, of looking after your delegates, greatly helps the success of the entire project.

The final programme

The first important decision regarding the final programme is to be quite sure which committee members are responsible for writing the different sections. Copy must be in press by the two-month mark at the very latest. Ideally, the final programme should be pocket size—15cm × 25cm—and should contain information about the outline programme, including both the social events and scientific programme, in both French and English; and general information, also in French and English, consisting of:

- *Registration and information centre*: location and times of opening and telephone numbers;
- *Congress secretariat*: as above;
- *Congress badges*: explanation of various colours where necessary;

note on procedure should they be lost (that is, report to secretariat immediately); and, most important, the request that badges should be worn at all times (see note on security);

• *Press office*: location, telephone, and opening times; the press office should handle all requests for interviews, press conferences, and photographs;

• *Trade exhibitions*: location, opening times, time of official opening ceremony, and telephone number of trade information desk; a large section of the final programme will, of course, be devoted to the trade exhibition, which will give a complete list of all firms attending, their stand numbers, and a profile of their products;

• *Travel bureau*: location, opening times, and telephone;

• *Airline office*: as above;

• *Banking services*: as above;

• *Post office*: A postal and telecommunications service should be provided for delegates from a temporary post office located in X area. The post office will be open from 0900 to 1600 hours, and its telephone number should be given. Outgoing calls may be made from public telephone boxes located at 1, 2, 3, 4 points. The cost of a local call is Xp;

• *Refreshments*: location, opening times, and approximate prices. Continental people do not have the same drinking habits as the British and providing special lunch bars and beer tents is not a viable proposition. Nevertheless, a bar accommodating about 200 people, open all day and situated in the trade exhibition should be adequate. Remember that to have your own bar in, for example, university premises does not absolve the committee from responsibility for finding out if special licensing permission must be obtained;

• *Medical services*: in cases of emergency the usual facilities would be available, but with a conference held within a university it is a good idea to cooperate with the university medical service, which has regular consulting hours and a resident dental staff. These facilities can be announced in the final programme—do remember to obtain official blessing from the director of the university medical centre;

• *Taxis*: telephone numbers of main taxi firms in the area;

• *Self-drive car hire and chauffeur-driven cars*: as above;

• *Public bus services*: details of main city services to and from conference centre;

• *Family social programme*: location plus full details of programme;

• *Maps*: pull-out maps of city centre and conference area; don't forget to clear copyright where necessary;

- *Scientific programme*: give full details;
- *Advertisers*: advertising is an important source of revenue and should greatly defray the costs of producing the final programme. A committee member should be delegated to sell advertising space, or you may choose to employ the services of an advertising agent. We recommend you do the job yourself. An agent charges commission, often payable also to other subcontracted agents, and is quite likely to omit many local advertisers whom a committee member could easily contact.

Temporary staff

In a large meeting you may need up to 40 temporary staff divided equally between medical students, who should be responsible for slide collection, and arts students, who can act as stewards and interpreters in the registration area. The arts students may be helped by members of the local Women's Royal Voluntary Service, especially for coping with inquiries regarding the city and local districts at the information desk at the time of registration.

The languages that we think it is essential to cover are French, German, Italian, Spanish, and Russian. French is the second language of many delegates from the Middle East and from Eastern Europe, and Spanish speakers are appreciative if, after a journey from South America, they are not obliged to speak English.

It is well worth having a safety margin in your staff numbers, as well as having enough people to cover for lunch and coffee breaks, it is essential to have people "on hand" to accompany delegates in special circumstances: for example, to retrieve lost luggage at the railway station or airport, or to accompany someone to the hospital casualty department. To be able to provide a certain amount of handholding makes the important difference between delegates feeling that they have arrived, and feeling that they have arrived and can now relax.

Official receptions

You will certainly have to arrange at least one official reception. These are some of the considerations in staging an opening ceremony:

Hall

Book the hall from the city two years in advance. Ushers and floral

189

decorations may well have to be arranged through separate suppliers.

Public address systems

A special contractor may have to be engaged, but obviously you cannot discuss these requirements until you have made final plans for placing your platform party.

Platform party

Who receives them on arrival at the hall? Check the order of precedence for city dignitaries in the line-up. Order of speeches? Drinks before, after, or both?

Refreshments

If refreshments are being provided for participants, check on the licensing laws and local rules; for example, no alcohol may be sold in certain halls booked for an opening.

Orchestra

Some entertainment before the ceremony is much appreciated. A concert goes down well, but you will have to book the orchestra a year in advance. Do not forget that if your concert is broadcast live or taped for broadcast you may receive a considerable reduction in the usual fee charged by the orchestra.

Official invitations

Be quite clear among committee members about who will receive official invitations to attend receptions, and whose task it is to issue these invitations. Also, do not overlook the ease with which it is possible to forget that tickets must be printed for such events, including special tickets for the platform party.

Programmes

Don't forget that, once the programmes are printed, you still have to arrange to have them distributed.

Flowers

Floral decorations are needed for the stage at the opening ceremony at least, but don't forget that a display of flowers in the registration area or trade exhibition enhances its appearance. All major cities have a parks and gardens department and it is often possible to rent flowers from such bodies.

Umbrellas

In the UK, at least, it is wise to have a few large umbrellas available at the entrance to your receptions, and people there to carry them. Indeed, some meetings produce umbrellas with the conference logo on them, for sale at a profit.

Transport

If special transport is provided for your delegates, do remember that in the UK it is illegal to take payment for a fare or to issue tickets on a hired bus.

Taxis

Tell local taxi services about the time and location of your special functions: a queue of taxis by a concert hall exit can do no harm.

Public relations/press officer

The public relations and press management of any conference are specialist jobs. The university press officer may make you this kind of offer; failing this, make quite sure that one person, and one only, is delegated as press officer. The following are intended as guidelines on how to approach the subject, but your first step should be to form a small public relations committee consisting of, say, four or five members, including representatives from the local press.

Advance publicity

At four months from the start of your conference, invitations should be sent by your public relations officer to the national press, TV, BBC radio, and local radio stations, as well as to editors of the professional and trade press, inviting them to attend, or, if they wish, make arrangements to cover the conference. The invitation letter should be accompanied by a press release giving the date, location, countries attending, and an outline programme. This information should also go to the Commonwealth Press Union; Press Association; Reuters; Foreign Press Association; and US correspondents in London.

At this stage the press office should compile profiles of newsworthy delegates attending the conference and any items of particular interest in the scientific programme or trade exhibition.

Advance press conference

Late during the week before the conference, the main office-bearers should take a press conference attended by visiting journalists, national and local press, TV, BBC and local radio—all invited to attend by the public relations officer. This press conference should cover the whole ground of the following week's proceedings.

Publicity during the conference

The press are invited to attend the opening and closing ceremonies, all appropriate scientific sessions, and all social events and receptions. Evening press conferences may be arranged at the end of each working day in the press office, where the chairpersons of the various sessions can give an account of the day's proceedings.

Press office

A temporary press office should be set up in the conference centre, consisting of the working press office itself and a room suitable for press interviews and sound radio interviews. The office should have available all morning national papers; all current press releases; advance copies of speeches; copies of congress programmes; general literature on the societies taking part; and refreshments.

The press office should be set up two days before the delegates arrive and should operate until the final press conference has been held.

Press cards

These must be available for distribution to press members.

Insurance

The following insurance cover must be taken out by the local organising committee:

- *Public and employer's liability* This covers injury or damage to, or caused by, committee employees. It is inexpensive but essential—indeed, a legal obligation. Cover for £1m can be arranged for a modest premium.
- *Abandonment cover* This figure must equal the irrecoverable expenditure that would be incurred by the committee were the conference to be cancelled at the last minute—due to strikes, fires, epidemics, and so on. It must also include such unpaid commit-

ments as perishable stocks laid in by caterers for events that have to be cancelled.

● *Briefcases* These will certainly have to be stored on conference or committee premises, for a few days at least. Make sure you insure against their loss by fire or theft.

● *Office contents* No matter how modest your office, or how many of its contents are borrowed or lent, take out an "all risks" policy to cover its contents.

Finally, check that the number of people you intend to accommodate in the various halls and lecture theatres does not contravene local fire regulations. Fire regulations are surprisingly strict and neglecting them could be disastrous.

Security

Unfortunately, it is a fact of life that large gatherings of people (especially in a confined space) attract the criminal element of any community, especially petty thieves. It is therefore essential that a security service be provided. The university security officer can often provide a first-class 24-hour service to cover all conference premises. It is extremely important that delegates should always wear their conference badge. People not wearing a badge should be asked by a security officer to identify themselves.

Cleaning

Special cleaning services will have to be arranged for conference premises, including the trade exhibition. Little things like unemptied ashtrays create a bad impression. The best and obvious source of the service is the body from whom you rent the premises.

Office equipment

Temporary telephones

British Telecom requires a week's notice to install temporary telephones. Be particularly careful about telephones. *Visit* everyone concerned in providing the service and be on hand to go round the actual location with the installation engineers. Temporary telephone numbers appear in your final programme and they must be correct. It is unbelievably easy to get them wrong. Check each on site. Temporary telephones are necessary but expensive.

193

Photocopiers

Your secretariat will require a photocopier from the word go, and the press office will almost certainly need one during the conference. These can be obtained on a short-term rental and you may be able to obtain more favourable terms by renting through your university or hospital.

Spare typewriter or word processor

A remarkable number of delegates will ask for typing facilities, so have a spare typewriter or word processor for their use.

Attendance certificates

A popular request, so have them prepared in advance with nothing to complete but the delegate's name.

The social programme

The social programme and the arrangements for entertaining the spouses of delegates are subordinate to those of the main meeting, but their importance should not be underestimated. Get the registration right and get the family programme right, and the conference will succeed. From the outset one member of the organising committee should be charged solely with this duty, and the committee must decide early on the general form of the entertainment and how much they wish to spend on it. The form is largely determined by the length of the meeting, the custom of previous occasions, and the requirements of protocol. The aim is at entertaining the delegates and their families and, while you should not rely too heavily on inspired improvisation or the natural generosity of the hosts, there is room for imagination and the light touch.

The main events of the social programme normally form a pattern. There is an opening ceremony, receptions, a show or stage performance, a free evening, and a dinner. Closing the conference is usually a modest affair at the end of the business programme. The social programme should not be a major item in the budget. Comparison with previous meetings may help you to decide the level of entertainment. Receptions are usually provided by the civic authorities, university, or local professional bodies. Such potential hosts should be contacted as soon as possible and the tentative dates and maximum numbers established. Large formal dinners are much more expensive than they were a few years ago, and individual attitudes to them vary so much that the dinner, which is usually the last formal social event, is costed separately and paid for by ticket. The main expense of the social programme lies in the opening ceremony. Whatever else fails, the opening ceremony must succeed—so that the available money should be concentrated on this. The possibility of arranging an opera, concert, or theatre performance will, of course, vary from place to place, but in general it is much cheaper to arrange block bookings for scheduled performances than to stage something special. The latter is really possible only if the state or civic authorities will meet the cost.

Some general points

Most of the social programme is in the evening. The timing of events will depend on that of the conference programme but must allow for delegates returning to their hotels to change and dine. A firm decision should be taken about dress at the various functions and advice about this included in both the preliminary and the final programmes. Availability of transport at night must be borne in mind. If there is an official conference photographer, he or she should be expected to attend the main evening events, but freelance photographers should be discouraged.

Besides the main events, the committee must think of the facilities available on the conference site. Registration for a large international meeting is a lengthy business, and delegates tend to loiter in the reception area in the hope of meeting friends or making sure that their arrangements are complete. Some lounge accommodation with coffee, and a desk dealing with social events ease the handling of large numbers. The questions of lunch for delegates, bar facilities, and hospitality rooms are matters for the main committee, and are best considered with the arrangements for the business part of the meeting.

The opening ceremony

The opening ceremony is attended by most of the delegates and their spouses. It is an opportunity to invite local dignitaries and those who have helped with the organisation. It is an occasion for the press. The numbers are large and may demand a hall larger than anything on the conference site. Think big. Spare seats may be filled by enlarging the circle of friends or by judicious advertisement. If the opening is to be a large affair, it is probably most conveniently

195

held in the evening of the day of registration, before the start of the conference proper. The time will depend on local custom and the hour of dinner in local hotels. Since the ceremony is a form of entertainment, it will last two hours or so, and speeches should be kept short.

Start the evening with a short display or concert lasting 40 minutes. Allow 20 minutes to assemble the platform party and reset the stage. The formal speeches need take no longer than an hour. Their number and order will be decided by the main committee according to protocol. The necessary mood of relaxed anticipation may be prolonged if a wine buffet is in prospect at the end of the evening. Arrangements include signposting the hall, since it may not be on the conference site, arranging flowers in the foyer and on the platform, ensuring that there is adequate transport for delegates to and from the hall, and notifying the police for security and control of traffic. Finally, it is worth considering employing an official master of ceremonies who will be responsible for the platform party and introducing speakers for this occasion.

Receptions and free evening

Receptions and free evenings are no problem, since the hosts will deal with the detailed organisation. The limiting size seems to be about 300 guests, so that it is convenient, at a large conference, to disperse the party among several simultaneous receptions. All that the social committee will have to do is to allocate guests to each, and arrange transport.

It is a great advantage, especially in a large international meeting, to leave at least one night free of formal entertainment. There may well be local delegates who will welcome the chance to repay hospitality and there are often sectional interests within the main conference—regional clubs, class reunions, and the like—that may use the occasion. The latter may be glad of a little space on the printed programme and may ask for a desk in the registration area or a hospitality room.

Hospitality rooms, social club, family club

The question of hospitality rooms arises only at large conferences: they are rooms at or near the registration area where important visitors may be entertained in some comfort, or conference business transacted. The number of hospitality rooms should be kept to a minimum, usually restricting their use to the chairperson of the organising committee, the president of the conference, and the press. The rooms should be clearly signposted and should have telephones.

Catering for lunches, a social club, and a family club, are all related and depend on the size of the conference and existing local services. Modern conference centres may take account of all this but where a purpose-built centre is not used, it is still important to keep all aspects of the meeting as close together as possible. Ideally, the registration area, restaurant, lounge, and bar should be in the same building. Where this isn't possible, the catering should be close to the venue of the meeting. If the conference is being supported by a trade exhibition, the lounge and bar may be sited close to it to attract delegates to the exhibition. When everything can be centred on the registration area there may be no need for a family club but, if one is to be provided, the relevant committee must decide whether it is to be near the conference site or near the town shopping centre. There are advantages in both.

The family programme

The family programme includes a range of entertainment for the spouses of delegates and, indeed, anyone who wants a day off from the meeting. Some of this can be organised professionally: conducted tours of the city or bus tours of the surrounding countryside. But there are questions of home hospitality, coffee parties, and a family or ladies' club, which can be dealt with by a separate committee. At an early stage, it is a good idea to choose a convener of this committee, who can discuss with the organising committee the dates, expected numbers, whether or not a family or ladies' club will be needed, what should be organised by the committee and what by official travel agents, and what money will be available for a family programme. Once these main lines are clear, the convener can organise a small committee to be responsible for the details and which, much nearer the time, can mobilise such local support as is needed. Arrangements for a family programme have to be rather tentative, because the number of visiting spouses remains uncertain until registration, but it is wise to overestimate, especially in calculating numbers for bus tours. Again, during the conference itself, it is better to mobilise too many of the "home team" than too few, as this spreads the load more comfortably.

The family programme should be scheduled during the hours of the main meeting, evening events being poorly attended. Bus tours are always popular. Fashion shows and similar displays are popular only if they relate to national dress or customs. Attendance at a conference can be fitted so easily into a package holiday that delegates may be accompanied by their whole family. It isn't necessary to organise a crèche, but it is worth collecting some information on how to amuse teenagers during the meeting and, indeed, the ladies' committee can help with the production of the printed conference brochure by compiling a list of useful telephone numbers and addresses of shops, taxis, hairdressers, and restaurants (graded according to cost of a meal).

The dinner

The dinner is the most difficult part of the programme to arrange—at least for a large conference. The problems are mostly related to the numbers of guests, and our discussion assumes a meeting of 1000 or more delegates. You can confidently predict that not all will attend the dinner. You may have some information about numbers at previous dinners but, even if only half attend, there will be too many for any hotel not built with an eye to the conference trade. This means using a hall not originally designed for catering and employing a firm of outside caterers. The success of the dinner will depend very largely on the latter, so they must be chosen with care. Use an established firm that is known to be capable of handling the expected numbers. Book them early, settle the venue of the dinner, and get an estimate of the cost per head. Wines form much of the cost, and you can save a lot by buying the wine in bulk as soon as possible to offset inevitable price rises in a year or two before the conference takes place. Any surplus wine can be sold at a profit after the event, so that this is a reasonable speculation.

Common sources of complaint are: too long an interval before dinner is served; slow service letting dinner get cold; not enough wine; inaudible after-dinner speeches. These difficulties arise from handling large numbers of guests. The pre-dinner interval should not be more than 45 minutes, but this time will be needed for the guests to arrive and sort themselves out, and to marshal top-table guests. Generous space should be allowed for foyer and cloakrooms, and plenty of extra cloakroom staff engaged. All wines, including drinks before dinner, should be included in the price of the ticket. It is courteous to meet top-table guests in the foyer and entertain them separately before dinner. It also ensures that they can be seated expeditiously in their proper places.

A big dinner demands a good toastmaster. His first duty will be to announce dinner. For very large numbers an individual seating plan is too laborious, but some sort of order must be imposed. One solution is to give out numbered cards on arrival, each matching one in the dining hall indicating a table or group of tables. The toastmaster can then invite the guests in to dinner by these numbers. Slow service and cold food are due to an over-ambitious menu with too many hot dishes. The first course—paté or hors d'oeuvres and a glass of sherry—can be on the table at the start. A hot soup can follow this, and then a cold main course with hot vegetables if desired, and a sweet and fruit to follow. A menu of this sort simplifies the choice of wine and lets the wine waiters concentrate on seeing that everyone is well served.

A short interval may be necessary between the end of dinner and the speeches. At a very large dinner it is unwise to announce this formally—it may be difficult to persuade the company to resume their seats. Speeches should be brief, clearly announced by the toastmaster, and audible throughout the hall. This means more than usual attention to the position of amplifiers throughout the hall. The toastmaster must be able to obtain silence for the speaker, who, in turn, may reasonably expect to be heard by everyone. The acoustic problems of large halls are often difficult and should not be left until the last minute. It is worth spending extra money to get an expert rather than an enthusiastic amateur, to arrange this.

One last word. Of all the conference papers, the dinner menu —dogeared, wine-stained, signed illegibly by old friends and new —remains the most durable souvenir. It should start the evening as a pretty thing.

Acknowledgments

The idea for these papers on how to organise an international medical meeting came from the happy association we had with the other members of the organising committee of the Joint Congress of the International Surgical Society and the International Cardiovascular Society held in Edinburgh in 1975 under the stimulating and provocative chairmanship of the late Sir John Bruce. We acknowledge the overall contributions made by Mr George A Hendry, the organising secretary of the Joint Congress; Mr William Reid, treasurer; Mr John McGhee, public relations officer of the City of Edinburgh; Mr Andrew Hay; Mr John Ward; Mr John Cook; and Miss Hannah Harkins.

Capperauld I, Reid W. Finances of a large international conference. *Journal of the Royal College of Surgeons of Edinburgh* 1976; **21**: 302.

27 Achieve success in international specialist meetings

J. Alexander-Williams, L P Fielding, S Goldberg,
R H Grace

The organisation of international meetings is a growth industry. Throughout the world individual organisations and cities compete, often ruthlessly, for the privilege of hosting such meetings. International specialist meetings provide a forum for the widest possible exchange of ideas on a narrow subject, ideas that may stimulate constructive criticism and mutual benefits among experts who might not otherwise meet. In this paper we propose directions for a successful specialist meeting and, in particular, introduce new ideas for communication. Our thoughts are based on extensive experience of attending such meetings, both good and bad, informative and boring, and, more immediately, on the experience gained by two of us (JA-W and RHG) in organising a medium-sized international meeting with 420 registrants in Birmingham in 1989 and by the other two (LPF and SG) in assessing it critically. We are aware that our experience and recommendations are relevant only for meetings of a similar size. Larger meetings attracting 1000 or more registrants have different rules, but we think that many of the principles defined here are still pertinent. We do not claim to have found the answers; all that we have been able to do is understand some of the questions.

We began the study by trying to define the purpose of an international specialist meeting; we then attempted to put these ideas into practice by running a meeting; and, finally, we held a postmortem examination to find out where the meeting had succeeded and where it had failed to achieve the objectives as defined in the purpose. Whatever the specialty, the aims of international meetings are similar and the problems are the same; our experience relates particularly to the specialty of coloproctology.

Purpose

Education is the main purpose of any scientific specialist meeting. Communication is needed to achieve this. Participants must have the opportunity to be exposed to new ideas and to question current conventional wisdom. Verbal communication among participants allows them the opportunity to question work that otherwise would be presented only in print. The probability of direct questioning in public should concentrate the speaker's mind and ensure honesty in presentation of data. Vulnerable data, when challenged, will be seen to be frail. It is at such meetings that "next season's" men and women will appear and thereby have an opportunity to enhance their career. It is by observing the performance in public of young research workers that future panellists are selected and lecturers overviewed. Conversations in corridors at such meetings often determine the direction of the career development of talented young trainees; this must be the lifeblood of the advancement of the specialty as much as that of the specialists.

Finance

Many meetings are financed largely from the advertising revenue of pharmaceutical, equipment, or service industries, and this has the danger of injecting commercial bias and may not be a permanent feature of future meetings. The financing of any international meeting depends partly on the registration fees of the participants. The more delegates attending, therefore, the more financially stable is the meeting and the more can be spent on the organisation. The travel budgets of many hospitals, institutions, and universities are limited, and financial support to attend the meetings is usually restricted to those who present data. Therefore, when selecting proffered papers there is an immediate dilemma between quality and quantity. There is conflict between the need to encourage the maximum number of delegates to attend to ensure financial stability and the need to maintain a high quality of individual presentation. We believe that quantity and quality are compatible only if all the presentations are subject to public criticism; no presentation should be hidden in the meeting merely to encourage attendance. We disapprove of the practice of having papers accepted under the euphemism "read by title" or having posters that are not subjected to criticism. Three of us (JA-W, LPF, and SG) have participated in a highly successful world congress of gastroenterology in Sydney, where there were over 6000 registrants. With that number it was clearly not possible to have every delegate's proffered work subjected to peer review as open criticism, and most delegates could have their attendance sponsored only if their work was accepted. The pragmatic solution was to publish those abstracts that were accepted but not selected for open discussion as a podium or poster presentation. They were published in a book the size of a respectable telephone directory but were never discussed. Delegates were invited to display enlarged versions of their abstract as posters that were not staffed or discussed. This compromise helps delegates to obtain sponsorship but is difficult to justify intellectually, as almost all abstracts are accepted and none criticised.

Is there no other way? Perhaps delegates should be sponsored only if they guarantee to pose an intelligent question in discussion time. Meetings with a reputation for quality will always attract delegates; such quality meetings held in an attractive venue will guarantee good attendance.

Use of time

All meetings have a time limit. The programme is planned within this limit, remembering that a plenary lecture of half an hour takes up the same time as three podium presentations or 10 poster discussions. Two parallel sessions allow twice as many presentations, but this has the disadvantage that participants cannot attend all presentations.

Methods of communication

Several of the ways of presenting information at meetings are discussed below.

State-of-the-art lectures

The state-of-the-art lecture usually honours a distinguished colleague or a great innovator. The speaker must have something to say, know the subject, and speak well; without these three principles there is no place for a formal lecture taking up so much precious time. We suggest that such lectures should be limited to 20 minutes.

Round table or panel discussion

The round table or panel discussion usually takes between one and two hours, with invited experts discussing a particular theme. We believe 90 minutes to be optimum and two hours too long. Members of the panel should be invited because of their particular expertise and their skill in argument. Sadly, they are sometimes asked because they are known to be eccentric or simply because of their seniority. The objective of such a panel should be to give an opportunity for divergent views to be aired and to allow the audience to hear experts expounding their point of view; in particular, arguing the merits of different opinions. The principal problem with such a round-table discussion is the variable quality of the experts and the limitations of their skills of communication. It is often difficult to keep senior experts to their allotted time or make them stick to the theme that is being developed. Brilliant panel discussions usually depend on the personality and communication skills of the moderator. In our experience international panels often fail to make the desired impact because members simply present a succession of expert papers, which are inexpertly delivered, on a succession of loosely related subjects. The presenters often overrun their time and thereby preclude useful discussion.

Panel discussion should be constructed so that opposing views are aired with ample time for interpanel and audience participation. The moderator must work hard well before the meeting, planning details and giving precise instructions to the panellists. The panellists should know the details of their copanellists' presentations, particularly their views on any points of controversy. Arguments add spice to a panel, but panellists perform better in arguments if they are forewarned of the controversy. We believe that the best panels are those in which the moderator asks the panel members to answer some previously circulated questions requiring short answers. Also, the moderator should allow the audience time to question and comment. This prearranged format requires meticulous preparation, with the chairperson and the panel members being aware which of the questions is their principal responsibility. It is often difficult to predict accurately the timing in such a panel. The chairperson should therefore leave the less important questions to the end so that he or she can stop and sum up before the scheduled closing time without having to rush at the end. Panels should end on time with the audience thirsting for more.

Original papers

Podium presentation

Podium presentation has always been the mainstay of any meeting. The organising committee has to decide how long should be allowed for individual presentations and how best to allow audience participation. In the past some meetings have allowed up to 20 minutes for each presentation, but recently 10 minutes has come to be accepted as the standard. With the expertise of presentation now expected, this could possibly be reduced to 8 minutes; 5 minutes for presentation and 3 for discussion. Presenters should not spend the first minute or two congratulating the committee on their wisdom in selecting their paper nor waste time with pompous presentations or facetious introductions. A short time limit should prevent insensitive enthusiasts presenting their life's work illustrated by a flurry of slides.

There is a tendency to group presentation on a similar subject together. This has the advantage of allowing the audience to concentrate on their subject of interest without having to move from hall to hall. There is a disadvantage if the chairperson groups papers together with all the discussion at the end. This may have a negative effect on subsequent discussion, with the earlier papers often being ignored. All presenters should be given the courtesy of receiving comments and questions from the audience. A good chairperson will try to leave some time for general discussion at the end of each theme.

The mechanism for audience participation needs careful consideration. The dilemma facing the chairperson is how to organise discussion from the floor. The solution has tended to be different on either side of the Atlantic. In the United Kingdom it has been usual to allow members of the audience free access to a microphone to allow them to criticise or question the speaker. This sometimes results in lame discussion from an audience reticent to expose its limitations of knowledge in public. When it works well, it allows genuine critique and results in contributions that are of value both to the speaker and to the audience.

In the United States and some parts of Europe there has been a tendency for such freedom of audience participation to be abused by some members of the audience who, lacking inhibition and, often, sensitivity, try to monopolise the discussion by delivering their own supplementary, loosely related paper, sometimes even trying to illustrate it with slides. In the United States the countermeasure to this abuse of discussion time has been to allow questions only in writing. These are selected and then posed by the chairperson. This usually limits discussion to brief questions because few moderators have the time, ability, or inclination to digest and reiterate complex contradictory statements. A glib one-line statement or question is always likely to be the moderator's choice. Attempts by the chairperson to call for comments and questions from named, forewarned discussants is often contrived and usually obvious.

We believe that the United Kingdom system of allowing questions and comments from the floor ensures the best discussion; the chairperson must deal firmly with any abuse of the privilege. Discussion from the floor requires good microphone back up. Roving microphones may be needed if there is theatre-style seating. We believe it best, however, to have discussants line up at microphones in the aisles as this alerts the chairperson to the potential number and eminence of prospective questioners.

Poster presentations

Usually, the best abstracts are accepted for podium presentation and the next highest scoring abstracts for poster presentation. We believe that it is better to select for posters those data that are best displayed in simple graphic form. It is often difficult, however, for the selection panel to make such decisions on the submitted abstracts, and it is difficult for authors to think of their data as poster material.

Decisions have to be made as to how many posters to accept and for how long they should be displayed to allow sufficient time for the audience to view them. We believe that it is very important to ensure that posters are adequately discussed. The numbers to be accepted may be determined by the space available for display. In single specialty meetings, where most of the participants will be interested in all the subjects, they can be discouraged by the prospect of viewing too many posters in too short a time. As experienced poster reviewers, we find that our limit is about 30 posters an hour. The audience must have sufficient time to view the posters, but they can partake of refreshment, even a finger buffet, while doing so.

The traditional format for poster discussion in the United

Kingdom is for the author to stand by the poster at set times during the meeting with the audience free to visit and discuss. In America it is more common for invited mediators to take small groups around the posters and discuss them with the presenters. If the group is of more than 12 people it is often difficult to hear and discuss, and many groups discussing at once sound like playtime at school.

We thought that neither of these formats was effective, and at our international colorectal meeting in Birmingham in 1989 we arranged that time should be set aside for poster discussion with the whole audience. A chairperson assisted by two moderators ran the meeting, with each presenter in turn being allowed two slides projected side by side. The first slide was an overall slide of the whole poster (as a reminder to the audience) and the second presented the conclusions. The presenter stood on the podium and simply responded when questioned by the audience. The role of the moderators was to lead the discussion by criticising or congratulating not only the content of the poster but also the form of presentation. With this format we were able to discuss 20 to 30 posters in an hour and to ensure that no presentation was listed on the programme without being subjected to peer review in open forum.

Audience participation

One of the shortcomings of large international gatherings is the lack of opportunity for the audience to participate actively in discussion and exchange of opinions. This is particularly frustrating in specialist medical meetings, where most of the audience are fully-trained clinicians. Modern technology, in the form of an interactive keypad system connected to a computer and videographic display, enables the audience to participate and respond to questions and indicate whether or not they agree with the principal speakers. We used this system at our colorectal meeting to involve the audience and a panel of experts in making decisions about the investigations and treatment of a series of patients with complicated Crohn's disease. The case history was presented, the audience were then given the choice of different investigations that they could order, and later they were given choice of treatment options. When they had indicated their answer to each question by pressing the appropriate key on the keypad, the international panel of experts were asked to respond. After the experts had committed themselves, the video projector displayed the percentage answers from the audience. Then panel members holding different opinions from the audience argued their view or said why they thought the audience were wrong. Whenever there was a particularly compelling argument, the vote was taken again to see whether the audience had been persuaded to change their views.

The interactive keypad system ensures a lively discussion and, if it is run well, holds the audience's attention. It is expensive, however, because keypads have to be installed at each seat or desk and connected to a computer. Much preparation is required in carefully choosing suitable questions and formulating the questions to fit the format of a multiple choice examination question. We believe that this is a promising method of communication, particularly at the international meeting, when answers from different national groups can be compared by the computers. The question session should, however, last only as long as the audience's interest can be maintained.

Breakfast sessions

In most meetings there is rarely time to discuss difficult or interesting clinical problems. This need can be met by what is sometimes called a breakfast or "meet the experts" session. Discussion takes place during breakfast at tables 10 to 16; 10 is optimum, as it allows everyone to hear and participate. Each table has a chairperson and co-chairperson, who either introduce discussion on clinical problems or respond to questions from the audience, who raise their own problems. Our organisation had the chairpeople remaining at the same table each morning of the meeting while the audience moved to a different table each day. Usually this is a popular session with both moderators and participants.

Other considerations

There are many other important activities that need careful consideration and planning, including the social programme, accommodation, transportation, committee and official society business. Not least, the overall organisers have to consider the extent of the burden that it is fair to inflict on local organisers and how careful planning and accumulated experience can ease the burden. These subjects are no less important than the scientific sessions in the recipe for a successful meeting.

28 Organise a medical symposium for general practitioners

David J T Wright

Many local and regional medical meetings for general practitioners take place each year. They are often organised by general practitioners who have never done such a thing before, and there is little published advice available. This is a simple guide on how to do it and includes a suggested timetable.

General principles

Start early. Good speakers, rooms, and caterers get booked up quickly.

Make sure you use fixed income (such as sponsorship) for fixed costs and number dependent income (such as registration fees) for number dependent costs. If you do not, you may find yourself financially embarrassed.

As soon as you have produced your provisional programme, apply to your adviser in general practice or postgraduate dean for section 63 approval.

Make sure there is someone other than yourself to "front" the course on the day. You will need to be available backstage to sort out the inevitable hitches that will occur.

Theme and programme

Decide on the theme. You may have been given a very wide brief (for example, practice organisation) or perhaps no brief at all. The theme needs to be broad enough to allow for some variety of topics but narrow enough to keep the meeting focused.

Fix a date.

Produce a provisional programme. Sketch out time slots and pencil in topics to be covered, together with potential speakers. Try to get a balance between local and national (or international, if you can get them) speakers. Don't forget spots for opening remarks, summing up and questions, and remember to include breaks for coffee, lunch, and tea. Consider varying the sessions: films, quizzes, and small groups can be put round the standard lecture by an expert.

Contact your speakers (see below). Don't forget to ask those you have put down to chair sessions.

Revise the programme in the light of response from speakers. Sometimes they will want to talk about something slightly different from what you had in mind. If they do not want to cover a point that you think is important you will have to ask someone else to cover that particular aspect.

Finalise the programme.

Venue

Usually the venue will be your local postgraduate centre. Check with the administrator that the centre will be available and confirm maximum numbers. Any other venue will probably mean considerable expense, but possibilities include rooms or conference centres in hotels and, out of term time, schools or colleges.

Speakers

Contact speakers as soon as possible to confirm that they are available on the day you want and are prepared to talk on a subject relevant to your programme. Local speakers can often be contacted by phone, but national or international experts will need to be written to.

Confirm acceptance, whether it comes by post or phone, with a letter. Thank the speaker for agreeing to speak and confirm date, time, place, subject, length of talk, and fee. Mention what equipment will be required. Say that you will be writing later with details of the programme and (if appropriate) a list of topics you would like covered.

Once the programme is finalised, write to speakers again, enclos-

209

ing a map showing the venue and a copy of the programme with their spot underlined. Spell out the important points you want covered and mention areas of potential overlap with other speakers. At this stage ask speakers to confirm when they plan to arrive, whether they will need transport from the station or airport, and whether they will be bringing a guest. If they are travelling long distances, ask whether they will require overnight accommodation.

If there is a dinner in the evening you might want to offer the main speakers and their guests complimentary places. If so, invite them now.

Finance

There are three main sources of income: sponsorship (usually from pharmaceutical companies); section 63 funds; and registration fee. As an example of the sort of proportions to expect, the following is a breakdown from an actual meeting; sponsorship 53%, section 63 funds 8%, registration fees 39%.

Sponsorship can be sought through pharmaceutical company representatives. Most postgraduate centres have lists of representatives with contact addresses and phone numbers. If you contact the companies direct, they will usually respond by suggesting that their local representative visits you at the surgery. Make sure you get confirmation in writing from the pharmaceutical companies of the amount of sponsorship they have promised.

Put together a provisional budget as soon as possible. Principal costs will be: speakers' fees and expenses; printing; postage and stationery; catering, including room hire for evening meal; and your own expenses—don't forget these, particularly phone costs and travel. All of these costs are fixed, apart from the catering costs, which will increase as the number of people attending the seminar increases. It is very important that these attendance related costs are covered by the registration fee. If they are not, you might find yourself in the sad position of losing money because of your success. If, for example, you are breaking even with 60 people attending and if the registration fees are £10 but the actual cost of providing coffee, lunch, and tea is £12, then every extra registration will cost you £2. Don't forget that meals taken by speakers, their guests, and any staff helping with the meeting will have to be paid for out of the fixed funds.

All the pharmaceutical companies who sponsor you will want

recognition on the day. Usually they will want to set up a stand. Space for these can be quite a problem if you are relying on small contributions from several companies, and it needs to be planned carefully. Make sure that the programme contains an acknowledgment of the sponsorship you have received. As long as pharmaceutical products are not mentioned there are no strict rules about the wording. "We would like to thank [company name(s)] for their generous sponsorship of this meeting" or a similar wording would be acceptable. Also, ask the chairperson to encourage everyone to visit the stands as he or she sums up before each break.

Catering

You will know your maximum numbers early on, as they will depend on the venue for the meeting, so arrange day catering (coffee, lunch, and tea) for that number. Cut down later if necessary. The hospital may well be the best contractor to use, but you should get quotes from outside caterers as well.

An evening dinner may be more successful if it is held away from the hospital. Most medium or large hotels have a selection of dining rooms to suit gatherings of different sizes. You will have to estimate numbers. If the meeting is a regular event, ask people who have organised previous years' dinners what numbers to expect. Make sure that all places finally booked have been paid for in advance so that if people fail to turn up at the last minute you won't be out of pocket.

Choose the menu as early as you can and decide what you are going to do about drinks. Will there be a "free bar"?—make sure you set a maximum limit with the bar staff. Will wine be included in the cost of the meal or be an extra payable individually—try to get at least some wine included in the cost.

Consider a seating plan with a top table for VIPs and invited guests such as the speakers. People are happier if they know where they are going to be sitting, and it saves the undignified rush for tables. Always have a seating plan for large numbers (say, over 50).

Accommodation

Accommodation required by speakers should be arranged with local hotels and bookings confirmed in writing.

If people coming on the course ask you to arrange accommodation for them, you can simply give them the names of local hotels and ask that they sort it out for themselves. Your local tourist information centre can often provide lists of suitable places.

Publicity

The invitation that goes out to your target audience should consist of a covering letter, a copy of the programme, and an application form. The covering letter should explain who the meeting is aimed at and give an outline of the theme and topics to be covered. It should list all the speakers, together with their title and institution, and say whether or not the meeting has section 63 approval.

Give a deadline for applications. Even though most people will ignore it, it is useful to be able to quote when you really do have to turn people down because they are too late. It is also worth stating how many places are available, particularly if the numbers are restricted.

The application form should list options (such as symposium only, lunch, or evening meal) and costs, and should be drafted so that it is easy for applicants to indicate what combinations they require and how many places they need. Make sure it says to whom cheques should be made payable and where to send them.

National advertising is usually expensive. Advertising in local medical magazines would be much less expensive. Posters in postgraduate centres are worth considering, and circulars can be distributed through the channels described below.

Printing

It may be worth paying for professional printing rather than using the hospital or practice photocopier. Try to get a pharmaceutical company to pay for the printing and distribution costs.

When you have decided on the venue for the evening dinner, have tickets printed to send to those who have booked and paid for the evening meal. They are useful for defining the number of guests who have been invited or paid for and for stipulating what dress is expected.

Distribution

Family practitioner committees will send out your information to all principals in their areas, but the distribution tends to be

Timetable

Six or more months ahead

- Decide on theme
- Produce provisional programme
- Contact speakers and confirm availability
- Arrange sponsorship
- Find and confirm venues for symposium and meals
- Get quotes from and book caterers
- Confirm section 63 status with adviser in general practice or postgraduate dean
- Book and confirm any special visits and entertainment if required
- Book accommodation for speakers if necessary

Three to six months ahead

- Finalise programme
- Confirm with speakers and readjust programme if necessary
- Confirm sponsorship and arrange layout of stands, etc
- Finalise menus and catering costs
- Print programme, covering letter, application forms, dinner tickets

Two to three months ahead

- Send out application forms, programme, and covering letter
- Final confirmation and briefing with speakers
- Check availability of any special equipment needed

Four to six weeks ahead

- Send out second batch of application forms if necessary

Two weeks ahead

- Confirm "final" numbers with caterers
- Confirm arrangements for lunch (may need more than one sitting)
- Check table seating and arrangement for evening dinner
- Order flowers for evening dinner if necessary

Day before

- Get out cash for gifts and incidental costs

On the day

- Check equipment
- Check that section 63 forms are available
- Check that registration table is set up
- Check that pharmaceutical company reps are happy
- Welcome speakers (make sure refreshments are available)
- Be ready to sort out any problems that occur

infrequent. This method does not reach retired general practitioners or general practitioner trainees in hospitals. Postgraduate centres will send out copies to their local practices and will be able to supply general practitioner trainees as well. General practitioner trainees can also be reached by sending applications to course organisers.

The only simple way you can reach retired general practitioners is if they are still members of the local faculty of the Royal College of General Practitioners. The faculty secretary will be able to provide you with a printout on sticky labels of names and addresses of all members and associates. The BMA used to provide a similar service but no longer does so because of the constraints of the Data Protection Act.

Consider sending personal invitations to local medical VIPs, particularly if they are associated with the organisation for whom you are arranging the meeting.

Confirmation of bookings

As applications come in they need to be confirmed. Your postgraduate centre administrator should be able to do this for you. Letters of confirmation should include a map and tickets for the evening meal or any other special event, if required.

Equipment

Make sure any unusual equipment required by any of the speakers is available.

On the day check that the overhead projector, slide projector, video, and any other pieces of equipment are working. Do this early so that there is time to sort out any problems before the meeting starts.

Consider having someone available during the meeting to work the equipment.

Registrations

As people arrive they will need to be registered and given name tags. Your postgraduate centre administrator should be able to organise this for you.

Miscellaneous

Consider having flowers on the tables at the dinner.

Consider having stands other than the ones provided by the pharmaceutical companies for people to look at during coffee and lunch breaks, but only if they are relevant to your theme—for example, general practitioner computer systems demonstrations would be suitable for a practice organisation seminar.

Don't forget gifts for any particular stalwart helpers (especially the postgraduate centre administrator).

Many speakers don't ask for any specific fee. In that case, average out what you can afford overall and pay flat rates to all the speakers, whether famous or not. Some speakers might prefer gifts, such as book tokens, rather than money.

Don't forget to have section 63 claim forms available on the day. It is a nuisance to have to post them all afterwards.

29 Prepare for a foreign fellow

Lindsay J Smith, Catherine Marraffa

Having an overseas graduate visit your department can be a rewarding experience for everyone: you gain a fresh enthusiastic worker for research or clinical work and the visitor gains a broader experience of medical practice. However, some forward planning is necessary to ensure that you both get the maximum out of the stay. A lot of daily tasks that are a routine part of your life may be difficult or even intimidating for someone from a different background.

One of the most important facts to know early in your preparation for your visitor is his or her family situation. Your enthusiastic helpful colleague may be reduced to an unworkable state because of worry about housing, spouse, accommodation, and schooling for the children.

Preparation

You should try to agree on a draft protocol of proposed work early in discussions. This allows the establishment of a background reading list. Remember that the library facilities may not be as extensive as you are used to and that forwarding key articles will allow valuable reading to be performed before arrival. A timetable of meetings, including locations at which the research work may be presented, will aid in the overall plan of your visitor's stay. Organise the use of the hospital and, possibly, university library ahead of arrival.

Suggested documentation for a foreign fellow

- General Medical Council certificate
- Original or notarised copy of degrees and higher qualifications
- Own medical council's letter of good standing
- Reference from previous consultants at home (for locum work)
- Letter of medical insurance cover from original country (if doing private locum work)
- Letter of good standing from own bank
- Letter of reference from someone in the United Kingdom (for bank account)
- Original car insurance certificates and no-claims bonus certificates
- Letters from children's schools about years of education and standard of achievement at time of departure

---

Cultural aspects

It should be remembered that the British culture embodies a historical perspective that differs significantly from other cultures in attitudes to social relationships, politics, and religion. With the majority of the NHS workforce being female, attitudes may be deeply offensive to foreign fellows. Religious practices and holidays must be respected. Though it is difficult to broach such subjects, timely intervention can defuse potentially explosive situations.

Housing

It is always reassuring when travelling any distance to know that there is somewhere to stay at the journey's end. If at all possible make every effort to secure some accommodation, either temporary or permanent, for your visitor. Contacting the hospital personnel officer, nursing officer, or local council is a good place to start.

You should try to see the proposed accommodation yourself. Remember that what you would have put up with as a student or while working on rotation may not be the sort of place to call a home for 12 months or longer.

When inspecting accommodation, look at the location with regard to public transport to the hospital. Obviously, a reasonable standard of repair, adequacy of facilities, presence or absence of furnishing, and an adequate number of rooms for the family size should be taken into account.

Transport

You will need to consider whether the position that your overseas graduate is to fill will need a car. Posts such as community paediatrics and on-call rotas covering two physically separated hospitals necessitate a car. Does the doctor have a driver's licence that is valid in the United Kingdom? Will he or she need to have an international driver's licence before arrival? The address of the AA (Automobile Association) or RAC (Royal Automobile Club) will help sort out these problems. The cost of cars and which dealers are reputable are two of the most daunting areas on arriving in a new country. Some guidelines about local dealers and prices in your area would be most welcome.

Try to obtain local public transport maps, ticket information, and a local street directory to send to or have ready for your visitor.

Children

Visitors bringing their children have particular needs that are often overlooked by permanent residents. Child benefit is payable once the children are resident for six months provided that a parent has a national insurance number. Children will probably fall sick at some time, so the address of the local family health services authority for the names of general practitioners will facilitate finding a family doctor. Remember, you don't want to be peering down an auroscope at 5.30 on a Friday evening trying to decide what, if anything, is wrong. Advise the visitor of the local immunisation schedules in force.

The school terms, age at entry, and waiting lists vary around the country and may be significantly different from those overseas. A list of schools close to the hospital as well as booklets on starting school can be obtained from the local council or library. If you forward this it will allow visitors to plan schooling for their children and allow such matters as level of schooling and equivalent academic performance to be sorted out.

Does the hospital have crèche facilities or are there local child minders who can be recommended?

Salary and cost of living

With all the advice you are gathering, the important factor that your prospective colleague needs to know is how much he or she can

218

expect to earn and how much it costs to live. With the increasing use of so-called soft money for the funding of posts, the salary may be completely unknown. Avoid the embarrassment of your visitor having to ask how much the salary is by stating it early on. If you will be advising locum work at nights or weekends to top up the salary, send a set of current rates from both the NHS and a locum agency. Sometimes the locum agency will require a period of employment in the United Kingdom so that a local reference can be obtained. Inquiry about the likelihood of this in relation to the experience of your visitor can avoid the difficulties of a period without top-up funds. If your visitor is coming to an NHS post, letters documenting the years of experience in the particular field should be brought so that the correct grade can be determined.

Remind visitors taking up an NHS post that superannuation will be deducted automatically unless they specifically opt out at the start. It is usual to opt out for short periods of employment in order to free more cash each month.

A list of scholarships can be applied for before or after arrival as well as some guidelines on application procedures and requirements would be appreciated by your visitor.

Your visitor must obtain a national insurance number as soon as possible: money earned without a national insurance number is not subject to tax relief, so all earnings are taxed at the emergency rate. The visitor should apply in person as soon as possible to the local social security office rather than allow the hospital personnel office to arrange it. The loss of several months of tax relief could be decisive in daily living as well as taking several months or even years to claim back.

The cost of living varies enormously throughout the United Kingdom, and the impression obtained from visiting London can give a worrying, jaundiced view. A simple idea of weekly grocery bills and transport costs is a good basis for your visitor.

Banking

Given that you have found the funding and somewhere to house your visitor, the handling of money should present no problem. However, the high street banks are notoriously reserved about opening accounts and granting cheque guarantee cards and automated teller machine cards (for example, cashpoint cards) because of the lack of a credit history in the United Kingdom. Ensure that your visitor brings a letter of reference from his or her own bank. You may need to provide a covering letter explaining the doctor's appointment. Having to go to the local branch during working hours to get money for six months can place a severe strain on productivity. An easy way of bringing money into the country is a small amount of cash and a personal cheque in pounds sterling drawn in the doctor's name. This will be cleared in a few days whereas foreign currency drafts may take several weeks, placing a strain on resources.

Staying on

Depending on the origin and family background of your visitor, various visas will be required by the Home Office to allow a visitor to work. The most common is a postgraduate visa that allows the recipient and family to stay for up to four years. These are currently the last bastion of sexism, in that if a woman is granted the visa, her husband is not allowed to work at all. The wife of a postgraduate husband is allowed to do any work, so check on the family plans. Having a husband at home all day unable to work can generate a lot of tension.

You should document the duration of the post at the outset and whether an extension is available or likely. Currently, health authorities are recommending that no overseas visitor be given a substantive post within the NHS without full evaluation of his or her immigration status.

When visas need to be extended, visitors often ask for the day off to go in person to Lunar House in the London Borough of Croydon. Permission should be freely given, as the alternative is to send the passport by post and be without it for up to six months while it is processed. It is not a happy situation to be in a foreign country without your passport. The trip to Lunar House will last at least all day, as the Home Office struggles with several hundred personal applications a day. Advise your colleague to go early and take every piece of documentation he or she can think of.

Odds and ends

The weather, a perennial favourite joke, should be taken seriously. An idea of the sort of winter and summer temperatures as well as the sort of clothing that is necessary, especially at the time of arrival, should be sent.

Remember the voltage in most countries is 220–240, but if any equipment is being brought over ensure it can operate on 240 volts.

A list of places of worship around the hospital can save a search on the day.

Remember that letters to some parts of the globe can take several weeks by airmail and the delay should be anticipated. Inclusion of a facsimile number will allow rapid communication.

This may all sound a long and difficult list of things to chase. The temptation is to allow visitors to sort it out when they arrive. A little planning, however, will ensure that they arrive happy and able to give you their best. Another good idea is to invite them to your home after a few weeks: it can be very lonely if you don't know anyone in a new country.

Index